INTERNAL ELIXIR CULTIVATION

The Nature of Daoist Meditation

INTERNAL ELIXIR CULTIVATION

The Nature of Daoist Meditation

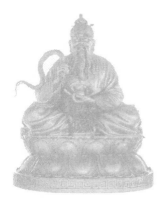

Robert James Coons

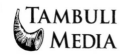

www.TambuliMedia.com
Spring House, PA USA

DISCLAIMER

First Published August 01, 2015 by Tambuli Media
Copyright @ 2015 by Robert James Coons
ISBN-10: 1-943155-13-5
ISBN-13: 978-1-943155-13-2
Library of Congress Control Number: 2015946737

Edited by Herb Borkland
Cover & Interior by Summer Bonne

FOREWORD

Robert Coons in an interesting individual. He is a Canadian who became enamored with Asian culture as a child, and later immersed himself in the traditional ways of China. He has studied areas as diverse as Daoism, internal martial arts, tea culture, poetry, calligraphy, brush painting, and pottery. And he is an expert in Daoist meditation, specifically the methods of cultivating the internal elixir, or life force energy; the topic of this book.

As a fellow traveler on the path of Chinese traditions including martial arts, traditional medicine and qigong practices, I have read several hundred books on the subject including contemporary works and translations of ancient texts. I was hoping to find a book on the topic to publish that would be fresh in its approach and clear in its lessons. I found these attributes in Coons' manuscript.

What makes *Internal Elixir Cultivation: The Nature of Daoist Meditation* special is the author's concise yet detailed approach to the topic. Unlike many works wherein the author seems compelled to shroud the content in enigmatic ideas and esoteric expressions, Coons instead uses direct, clear and simple language to teach the essence of the Daoist meditative method. In short, his work is deep and detailed, drawing on the most treasured ancient texts and teachings, yet at the same time is accessible and practical in its approach.

The work's editor, Herb Borkland, expressed the uniqueness of Coons' manuscript the best, when he wrote me the following sentences. "This is the work of an autodidact, and I bless his dedication and strength of mind and how he has digested and so can make legible so many elusive concepts. To use many words to advertise how to shut up is always the trap in meditation manuals. It seems to me he surmounts that paradox through a very Chinese quality of modest but unshakeable expertise."

And so Tambuli Media is proud to present to you Robert James Coons' *Internal Elixir Cultivation*, for which we are grateful to Robert Cory Del Medico for connecting us with the author. We hope you enjoy and benefit from this book as much as I have.

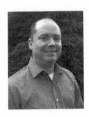

—Dr. Mark Wiley
Publisher, Tambuli Media

TABLE OF CONTENTS

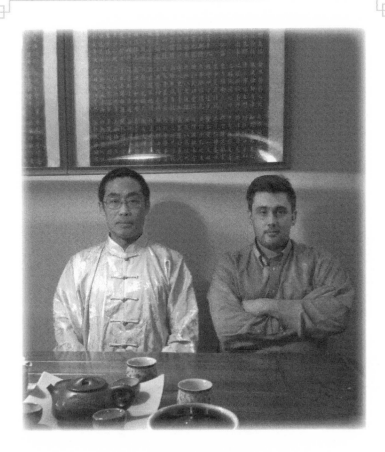

Robert James Coons and his teacher Yang Hai, seated in Master Yang's home in Montreal. Master Yang studied in the Beijing White Cloud Temple with Cao Zhenyang, abbot of the temple and leader of the Dragon Gate sect of Quanzhen Daoism at the time. He also studied in the Sanfeng lineage of Daoism and Tianjin, and with many other teachers who had Daoist teachings either passed down through family, or who had deep personal research into Daoist methods. He specializes in meditation, Chinese medicine, martial arts, qigong, knows various other Daoist arts such as face reading, and holds an MBA.

PREFACE

The West has come to a place of economic prominence in the world, leading to lifestyles which had never been imagined in the ancient world. People are now free to eat and drink whatever they wish – they are able to have access to the best health care and have the richest economy in the entire history of mankind. The West is the best it has ever been, and yet people feel a discord.

There is a lack of harmony in the physical and spiritual world of the western psyche—and although things are good, people are beginning to see that what they have gained in riches, they have begun to lose in spirit. People have also begun to feel the negative effects of a lavish lifestyle—with diseases such as addiction and mental illness at the forefront of society. Almost everyone has been touched by depression, anxiety, obesity, and severe emotional trauma and in the West today, there are very few people who are completely at ease and happy with their own lives.

There is a great move toward new ways of life, but it seems that there are too many roads and not enough maps. There are many promises of salvation, but almost none of them actually yield results.

People see the value in spirituality, but spiritual teachers are often more concerned with lining their own pockets or espousing political and cultural beliefs than with teaching people how to take control of their lives. Worse yet is the pseudo psychology of the pharmaceutical institutions, and the push for doctors to prescribe powerful drugs to people with simple-to-resolve emotional problems or even naturally-occurring states such as sadness. This is perverse and troubling. People are beginning to lose touch with their autonomy and to imagine that they have no control of their own lives.

It can be very difficult to find a good teacher; each practice has its own value. The special quality of Daoism is that the entire practice is laid out in the various meditation and philosophy classics that exist within its canon. With the guidance of a knowledgeable teacher and a good work ethic, students of Daoism may gradually improve their lives by learning to cultivate a feeling of inner awareness and understanding of how to accord with nature in a more harmonious and spontaneous way.

Although this knowledge is available in western religion and philosophy, it has mostly been lost over the racket of "buy now, pay as you go" style pop spirituality.

With the exception of orders such as the Jesuits, Christianity has basically lost its root in contemplative prayer. As such, many western people have begun to feel that the Christian doctrine is something which is taught to them rather than directly experienced. This has created a growth of interest among people in Eastern spiritual traditions such as Buddhism, Hinduism, and Daoism, but because these fields are still relatively new in the west, it is hard for people to contextualize all of the different facets of these practices. This leads to teachers coming forth and if not willingly cheating their students, at least, not being completely prepared for what the western student may face on the spiritual path. People often assume that meditation is a panacea and cure-all, so when they begin learning how to cultivate the practice, they often come to it with unrealistic expectations, and many people are let down and quit early. The meditation industry supports this type of behavior because although it is not beautiful, it is true that even spiritual teachers must put food on their tables, and, as such, many parts of the industry are quite reliant on making big promises in order to pull in new students. It is safe to say that nothing good ever comes to people who don't work for it.

The good news is the wisdom of past masters is still available, and people who wish to pursue the way of attaining the same wonderful benefits of meditation may continue to reap the benefit of a mindful practice.

Among spiritual cultivation practices, Daoism is a very special method. Daoism, although having a religious practice associated with it, is not constrained by the requirement of belief in any gods, prophecies, or proscribed methods of worship. Daoism works as a three part system, with each of the sections harmoniously operating together. Daoism is comprised of Daoist philosophy, religious practice, and meditation. Although it is good to know about each separate section of Daoism, it is also quite normal to specialize in one area of practice alone. Some people combine Daoist philosophy practice with meditation, while others combine meditation with religious practice. There is nothing wrong with that, and it is possible to make progress in Daoism even without believing in the religion.

I was fortunate enough to have followed a path of self-actualization from my early childhood. As a boy, my father, a teacher who was very interested in philosophy, religion, and science, gave me several books to read on the subjects of Daoism and Buddhism. Principally, he gave me, the *Tao of Pooh*, a children's book explaining Daoist philosophy, and *Zhuang Zi Speaks*, an excellent book by a Taiwanese cartoonist on the subject of the second great Daoist philosopher, Zhuangzi. The free and natural spirit of these books caught my imagination. It seemed as though the words jumped off the page and the open-hearted spirit of the authors made the spirit of their writing as plain as the blue sky. Zhuangzi especially writes in a very free and open way, suggesting that instead of imagining we know all of the answers of life, it is more useful to imagine that there are many things we don't know, and that we are always capable of learning and growing. From that time the long search for an enlightened life began.

Over the years, I encountered many spiritual sicknesses—bullied by my peers in school and always treated as an outsider. I grew withdrawn from normal children of my age. In my late teens, this culminated in a serious rejection of the public school system and a downward turn into a lifestyle of partying and wildness. It eventually culminated, at 19 years of age, when I had a serious accident that led to my hospitalization.

After that, I really needed to get my life on track and so began to search out new ways to understand both my relationship with the world around me, and also if there was a way to live a better and fuller life. I studied qigong, taijiquan, vippassana, baguzhang, xingyiquan, and many other modalities, but I found that the practice which always intrigued me the most was Daoist meditation. Daoism is a somewhat elusive practice in that it can be quite hard to find a teacher, and when I set out to find a good teacher, it took me quite a long time. I went to visit many different teachers in the internal martial arts, qigong, and meditation, and eventually did manage to find a great teacher who took me under his wing and shared many subtle and profound things with me.

Although it can be hard to find a teacher, there is still enough true Daoist practice remaining in the world for serious students to discover the real thing, so to speak. All varieties of spiritual practice have their strong and weak points, and each is suited to different personalities. That means that the truth which is contained in Daoism can also be found in Christianity, Buddhism, Islam, or any other type of practice which joins the mind of the practitioner with something larger than their own thoughts and feelings. I wrote this book for people who are interested in Daoism, and I hope that it will be useful and informative to help you start your journey into the very interesting world of meditation and spiritual illumination.

My journey started with a local Taijiquan teacher who focused much of her practice on obtaining internal quiet through qigong. Because of this, I was able to relieve some of the symptoms of my PTSD and to gain a feeling of calm and relaxation that I had not achieved since the time after my hospitalization. Naturally, I fell in love with the Daoist arts and wished to seek out the most genuine teachers with whom to study. The practice took me all over North America in search of great teachers—I had heard many stories of the seemingly magical skills of the ancient masters of martial arts and Daoism.

At the time, I was most interested in the internal martial arts of taijiquan, xingyiquan, and baguazhang and had read some excellent books, such as BK Frantzis' *Power of the Internal Martial Arts*, and the various books of Stuart Alve Olson, among others. The stories they conveyed of their own training, and stories of past masters who were able to defeat even the strongest opponents by only using four ounces of strength simply enthralled my young mind. Perhaps it was naïveté and lack of experience, but I thought of internal martial artists and Daoists as being somewhat like the Jedi in the film "Star Wars." It seemed like they could command their minds to defy gravity, and do things which were beyond the abilities of normal men. I had heard stories of people breaking huge piles of bricks with just their fingers, or running directly up tall walls, jumping along the lined roofs of houses. These high-level skills seemed so interesting, and in the world of Chinese martial arts, it is quite commonplace to venerate past masters by telling stories of their great achievements. This can be truly inspiring to beginner students as it shows some of the possibilities of these fantastic arts.

Eventually, I found two teachers who I feel really have the skills I so desired to learn. One was Peter Ralston, and although my time studying with him was admittedly short, his take on the world of the mind has always had an influence on the way I practice.

Peter works according to the philosophy of "not knowing." That is to say, much of his practice is focused around the art of remaining aware and conscious, rather than making assumptions about how a movement, an opponent, or the world should work. He teaches martial arts with a strong focus on developing the mind toward being effectively conscious. I truly took a great deal of benefit from his ideas as I progressed in the martial arts. I continue to use many of his concepts of relaxation and an open awareness as staples of my practice.

The act of being willing not to know something is the beginning of true honesty.

When people assume they know the answers to the problems which are presented to them by life, they stop themselves from really seeing the truth of what is going on. I have always respected Peter because he is able to convey to his students very directly that the ideal way to understand oneself is to remain open-minded and able to respond to situations as they arise, rather than simply creating a series of pre-programmed reactions to stimuli.

My other teacher, Yang Hai, a Chinese man from Tianjin who currently resides in Montreal, was the one who had the greatest impact on my study. He is a martial artist, a Daoist, and a Chinese medicine doctor who teaches according to the concept of unifying the tasks of everyday life so they may work harmoniously together. I learned more than martial arts and Daoism from him, but also how to live a more complete and harmonious life. One of his main principles can be summed up as "using culture and art to cultivate beauty." He believes that Chinese culture may be used as a spiritual cultivation system and allow people to reach their greatest potential: the potential to live a happy and long life. A good example of this is his grandfather, Yang Qinlin, who lived to be ninety-seven years old and practised martial arts and Chinese culture every day with great spirit and vitality, even up to shortly before he passed away. My teacher takes a great deal of his inspiration from these true Chinese gentlemen, who dedicated their entire lives to mastering themselves and attaining great achievements in the cultivation of health, longevity, and beauty.

Yang Hai is a family man, a spiritual cultivator, a master, and a student. I was so touched by his honest teachings on the subject of martial arts and Chinese culture that I took it upon myself to travel to China and learn the essence of China's 5,000 year old culture.

During the four years I spent in Shanghai, I became fluent in Mandarin Chinese, learned to read classical Chinese, studied tea, martial arts, painting, music, pottery, calligraphy, Daoism, poetry, and many other studies. My teachers are from all walks of life, and I have gone to places such as Beijing, Tianjin, Taipei, Tokyo, Sapporo, Fujian, Hangzhou, and Henan in order to seek out teachers and research this foreign culture which I have taken as my own.

At some point, it occurred to me that the knowledge which I have literally sweated, cried, and bled to learn may be of some use to others. I feel that although my accomplishment pales in comparison to my teachers', it has been of such great use to me that I must share it. I have gone from being a troubled young man with horrible symptoms of PTSD, such as night terrors, hallucinations, and affective schizophrenic tendencies, to a confident and happy person within the time of under a decade. I have made such a complete recovery that I feel as if I have been given a new life; and a large part of that life I owe to the practice of self-cultivation.

Were my path of cultivation some other art, such as yoga, I would now be writing a book about that; the first step on the path is the most important, and it does not matter which practice you choose, as long as you seek out competent teachers and study assiduously and without ceasing. It just so happens that the inclusive spirit of Daoism speaks to me, and as such, I have written this book. I suspect Daoism also speaks to you, so I hope that my words here will have a positive effect on your life and practice. If you work hard to understand the material presented in this book, you will also have a chance to develop a practice which can balance the mind and body, make you feel more healthy and dynamic, and help to clarify the thoughts in your mind into a more well-organized and productive way of understanding the world. As an adherent of the ethic of kindness, I would be remiss not to share the benefit of the insight I have gained through this lifestyle.

Many of the sicknesses of the modern world are easy to cure; most illnesses begin in the mind. People feel the pressure to conform placed on them by society; they are given stress in the workplace, home, and are constantly bombarded with information from the media. It seems like the modern mind is not allowed to rest, and so people are always wired on caffeine, sugar, or simply by their desire to perform according to expectations.

One of the ways the nervous system heals itself is through rest; and this is a lucky fact because the spirit of meditation is to allow the mind to rest. Essentially, there are two types of meditation, one which actively uses the mind to feel, and one which attempts to flick a dimmer switch on the consciousness for long enough that the body enters a state of deep tranquility and restfulness. Daoist meditations tends toward using the slowing of the thoughts as a way to cause the body to slow down and relax, thus allowing the parasympathetic nervous system to do the important work of regulating the hormones and repairing the body. Many of the true diseases of modernity, such as cancer, heart disease, and profound depression, can all be prevented and helped simply by following a healthy and happy lifestyle. Practicing meditation is a very good method to guard against becoming ill. Meditation allows the mind to become calm and the body to have time to reset itself. Sometimes a full night of sleep is not enough to heal the psychic trauma of the work place. In this situation, even half-an-hour of meditation each day can assist in allowing people to let their minds filter out the various stresses of their lives. I hope the practice presented in this book will allow you to take control of your mind, learn to relax, and give yourself enough time to heal.

Daoism as a practice is based on four basic concepts:

1) Embracing simplicity

2) Cultivating positivity

3) Nurturing energy

4) Retaining (not wasting) life's energy

Done with consistent practice, each of the exercises in this book embraces these basic virtues. The principles discussed here are not esoteric and they are achievable now, in this lifetime. In this book, I have laid out many of the best steps you can take to achieve this level of calm, clarity, and happiness. I think you will be able to learn my method quite quickly.

All of the great sages of human history were not great because they allowed people to live in ever higher realms of luxury. They were great because, to paraphrase the words of Jesus Christ, instead of giving a man a fish to feed him, it is better to teach him how to fish, thereby he may feed himself.

They themselves, who may have been poor in the physical realm, were rich enough in spirit to serve as lighthouses to guide others through the dark. People like the Buddha, Laozi, Christ, Gandhi, Nelson Mandela, and others underwent deprivation, taunting, and even risked their lives to help people on the path to freedom. I am not risking my life to write this book, and I am not a saint, but my goal is to do the small bit that I can to help extend the heart of righteousness and offer a helping hand to the people around me. I think the key behind the achievements of the ancient and modern masters is that they embraced the lives of others as being of equal important to their own. The teaching left behind by these compassionate spiritual teachers are all good, and all worthy of investigating. In this book, I will present what I believe to be a genuine shortcut to spiritual achievement. Daoism cuts out many of the filters of belief associated with religion and leaves behind principles which may be used regardless of one's affiliations or groups.

Although my spirit is not as well-developed as those of my teachers, it is my sincere desire to share with as many people as possible the benefit I have enjoyed through my studies.

Yang Hai once said to me that every day of his life feels like a holiday. At the time, I did not completely understand his meaning, but now, after a sufficient period of cultivation, I think I can say with clarity: the practice of calming the mind and developing spirit will make even the most stressed of people feel as though a great weight has been lifted from their chests.

The true benefit of Daoism is simply to become happier, and although happiness is ultimately in the hands of the individual, I think correct practice and a positive attitude can help people on the way to living happier lives. This book is a good primer in how to begin a correct practice. Daoist practice can provide people with time to reflect, to experience less interference from thoughts and emotions, and less attachment to desires. It is also a very good way to regain a sense of being rested and at ease in the world. These concepts are the foundation of the book, the premise upon which the reader will move into the next pages.

Although Daoist practice is not a panacea, it is a very good place to begin the study of achieving true happiness. The body and mind are inseparable, and if the state of the mind is full of the illness of stress, anger, fear, judgement, and hate, it will not be possible for the body to last long without also developing illnesses. People all have one primary responsibility which is more important than any other and that is to their own health. The belief of the Daoists is that once people have developed their health sufficiently, they should share with others. In this case, I am offering this book to you so you may also share the benefit of gaining in both happiness and a feeling of health, vitality, and well-being. The way of doing and understanding presented in this book can help to cure many of the stresses and ills inflicted by modern society and allow people to overcome many obstacles which may originally have seemed impossible. It is my sincere hope you will get as much benefit from this book as I have from the instruction of my teachers and my own practice.

THREE DANTIAN

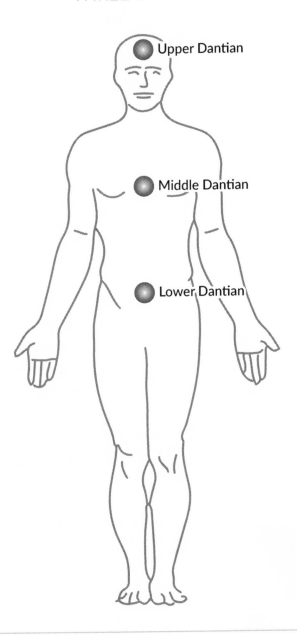

CHAPTER 1:

DANTIAN –
THE FIELD OF ELIXIR

Daoists believe that the universe is a great conduit of energy. This energy is known as *dan,* or elixir. *Dan* is said to pervade all things at all times and is the force which always nourishes the universe. Just as this energy exists in the universe, Daoists believe it exists in people, too.

During the early history of Daoism, the concept of dan is not clearly disseminated, but after several generations, Daoist theorists began to put together the idea that *dan* could pervade certain parts of the body and serve the function of feeding the organs and limbs with life energy.

Although early Daoism viewed *dan* as being a transferable energy that could be focused anywhere in the body, it eventually became known as primarily existing in three main parts of the body. These three parts are called *xia* (lower), *zhong* (middle), and *shang* (upper) *dantian.*

Most importantly, the lower abdomen is considered to be the seat of *dan* in the body. This area is not a specific one, but rather a general area that contains this elixir energy. Daoists believe it can be stirred and improved by focusing the attention on the lower abdomen and breathing calmly and slowly while gradually relaxing and feeling the gradual movement of the in and out breaths as they come and go.

The function of this part of the body is related to the concept that the kidneys and genitals are directly above and below the abdomen area. These two points are considered to be extremely important to the health of people over the course of their lives.

The genitals are associated with reproduction and creative power, while the kidneys are held to be representative of the ability of the body to clean itself. As such, the *dantian* between these two places becomes a centre where there is a great deal of vital activity taking place which can decide the health of an individual.

When considering modern science, it is quite accurate to say that the area around the lower abdomen is indeed extremely important to the overall function of the body and mind. Not only does the area contain the majority of reproductive and digestive organs, it also contains the majority of the sympathetic and parasympathetic nervous systems.

圖 胎 道

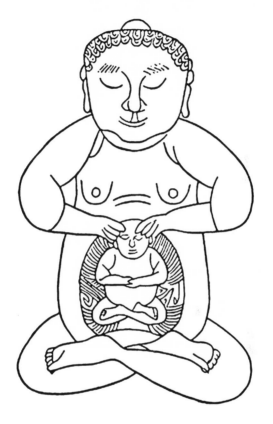

Cultivating the Embryo: Daoists often refer to cultivation of the Dantian as a method of creating a divine embryo in the body. Some people believe that when this embryo is mature, it can leave the body and travel the universe. This picture is taken from Wang Changyong's book "secret of the golden flower," a book on the cultivation techniques of the Northern school of the Complete Reality school of Daoism.

These two parts of the autonomous nervous system take care of functions such as "fight or flight," rest, sexuality, healing, and many other important things. They are also considered as not being consciously controllable by people, unlike the central nervous system, which to some extent can be felt and manipulated.

Daoists seem to have discovered that by simply focusing the mind and breathe on the area around the lower abdomen, they can indirectly assist the function of the autonomous nervous system and improve their health and longevity.

The other two *dantian* are located in the centre of the chest and head. The chest is considered to be associated with breathing and the heartbeat. The head is considered to be associated mainly with the function of the brain.

We will get to ways to practice with each of the *dantian* a little later in this book, but for the time being, why not sit back in a comfortable chair, feel yourself breathing in and out, and slowly place your mind into your lower abdomen, while maintaining a light focus on the breath.

DANTIAN BREATHING

The great master Hu Haiya told my teacher that the best way to learn meditation was to sit back in a comfortable chair and simply feel the breaths coming and going from the body.

- ❖ *Take a moment to sit down, lean back, close your eyes, and let the breath gradually come and go as it will.*

- ❖ *As you begin to relax, slowly place the feeling aspect of your mind into your lower Dantian and leave it there.*

- ❖ *If it moves, simply put it back, and don't force it to do anything else.*

- ❖ *Stay like this for a few minutes and simply notice how it feels to breathe and keep the mind in the abdomen.*

- ❖ *When you are ready, gradually open your eyes and massage your face with the palms of your hands a few times.*

- ❖ *Observe how you feel, and repeat this practice often in order to begin building a solid foundation of relaxation and awareness from which to work.*

THREE GATES

Yuzhen

Jiaji

Mingmen

CHAPTER 2:

SANGUAN SANTIAN –
THREE GATES THEORY

Daoism has a core concept which is based around how to cultivate the energy field of the universe in one's own body. As previously mentioned, *dantian* is used as a concept to illustrate how energy exists and moves in the body. The *dantian* are split into upper, middle, and lower, and in order to practice using the *dantian*, we can begin to focus on the inner abdomen while breathing naturally.

Before we can address how energy moves through the three *dantian*, we must first explore another concept called *San Guan*, or Three Gates Theory. The three gates of the body are said to be places which energy moves through but does not rest in. They are located in the back of the torso and begin at the coccyx, above the kidneys, and finally in the neck and occipital bone in the back of the head.

These three gates are called *ming men*, *jia ji*, and *yuzhen*, and each serves a different function in the transportation of energy through the body.

The *ming men* area from the coccyx to the base of the kidneys is usually related to the lower *dantian*, and one principle of Daoism is that when the mind is placed in the lower *dantian* for a long enough time, there will gradually be a sensation which begins to move up the spine. The route that it initially takes is from the point half way between the belly button and genitals, and then naturally manifests as a sensation of increased feeling in the spine, moving upward to the top of the head. This sensation first moves through the *ming men*, then the *jia ji*, and finally through the *yuzhen* and to the top of the head.

The movement of energy through the *ming men* is often explained as being similar in speed and strength to a galloping horse. When the energy arrives at the *jia ji*, it is said to feel more light and fast, like a deer running quickly through the grasslands. Finally, the energy moving through the *yuzhen* is equated to being like a slow and strong ox pulling a laden cart.

The concept of the three gates is the opposite of the *dantian* principle. While *dantian* store energy, the three gates may only transfer it. While the *dantian* may be focused upon during practice, Daoists believe the three gates are only active at an autonomic level, so it is not recommended to attempt to directly work with the three gates during meditation.

One way of thinking about the three gates is by considering their relationship with the autonomic nervous system. This system consists of the nerves which control unconscious aspects of the physiology of the body. It is comprised of two parts, one called the sympathetic nervous system, and the other known as the parasympathetic nervous system.

These two nervous systems control things like breathing, sexual function, "fight or flight" response, and rest and healing processes of the body. This two-part nervous system is the major aspect of the functioning of the brain which exists outside of the Central Nervous System. It mostly exists under the neck and in the lower part of the torso. This nervous system functions by itself, and for the most part cannot be consciously controlled.

One of the goals of Daoist meditation practice is to allow the autonomic nervous system to function better. By placing the mind into the lower *dantian* until energy moves by itself, it is possible to stop the mind from processing the majority of verbal thought normally occurring in the mind at any given time.

The lower abdomen is often considered to be a second brain, in that it serves many of the functions which control the physiology of the body. This brain, which is represented as certain aspects of the autonomic nervous system and endocrine system, is a non-thinking entity but has a large role in the processing of the brain as does the Central Nervous System and conscious activity.

I believe that this is the key reason why we place the intention into the abdomen during the meditation process. By doing this, we can allow the body to accord to its natural intelligence, rather than our own thoughts, which mostly occur as images, words, and feelings in our brains and manifest as emotional feelings in the heart or chest area.

Because focusing on the lower *dantian* will eventually cause the meditator to become more calm and relaxed, as well as cause more sensation to move through the back and spine, it is called the "Reverse Flow," in Daoism. This reverse flow is thought to be opposite to the normal manifestation of thoughts and emotions, which in Daoist thought normally move upward in the body and become stuck in the chest and head.

When we meditate on the lower *dantian*, we begin to allow this "stuck" energy to sink downward and clear out spiritual blockages caused by negative emotions.

When the energy suddenly rises through the three gates to the head, usually Daoists will simply observe the feeling and let the consciousness rest inside of the head, maintaining softness of breath and simply sit with the feeling until it begins to move again.

The feeling will eventually begin to sink toward the chest, and when it arrives completely in the chest, at this time they will simply breathe naturally until the feeling moves again, back to the lower *dantian*.

The biggest goal of this practice is to clear out energetic and spiritual blockages in the torso and head while calming the Central Nervous System and allowing the Autonomic Nervous System to do its job with less interference.

This topic will be further touched upon during the next chapter, discussing the *Zhou Tian*, or "Heavenly Orbit."

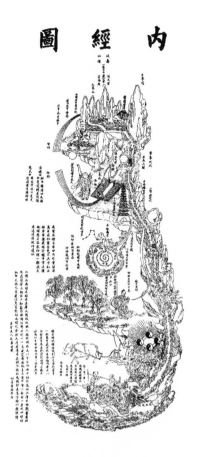

Neijing tu: The Nejing tu is a Daoist map of the energy body which shows in detail the alignment of the spine, head, upper, middle, and lower dantian, as well as the qi xue, point and various other details associated with meditation practice. The image of a mountain is used to explain the human body, with various different levels of the mountain being represented by different important aspects of the human energy body. The ox at the bottom represents the lower dantian and Jing energy, while the swirling aspect of the center represents the breath as it comes into the lungs. At the top there is a picture of the sun and a meditating Buddha, they both represent how the important energy anatomy at the top of the head relates to human enlightenment.

CHAPTER 3:

XIAO ZHOU TIAN –
THE MICROCOSMIC ORBIT

A key technical aspect of Daoism is the concept of *yuan qi*, or "the continuously flowing energy of the universe." This is the eternal nature of all things – a type of energy which always circulates without stopping. Daoists call this *zhou tian,* or "the continuous orbit of energy in the universe."

Daoists believe that the universe is a macrocosm of all living things and that living things are a microcosm of the universe—so all beings also contain a small version of the energy and spirit of the universe. As such, all beings are connected to each other by universal spirit.

Early Daoism developed at the end of the Eastern Zhou Dynasty—a time in which the earlier religion of the Shang dynasty had been replaced by the Zhou leaders' ideas about the creation.

The Shang dynasty rulers had believed in a god known as Shang Di, or "the great emperor"—a governor of all things in the world. During the Zhou dynasty, the emphasis was taken away from Shang Di and placed on a new concept called *tian di*, or "the emperor of heaven." This idea was based on the worship of universalism, as opposed to an individual god. Under this mandate, all things in the universe were taken together as one, with the Zhou dynasty ruler as the king of heaven on earth.

Laozi himself rejects the idea of a god, preferring instead to treat the universe as a neutral and non-judgemental creator which simply created and destroyed things through the cycles of nature rather than choosing to benefit certain beings over others.

> *The world is not compassionate,*
> *for it sees all beings as grass dogs,*
> *the sage is not compassionate,*
> *for he sees all men as grass dogs.*
> *The space between heaven and earth,*
> *is it not like a bellows?*
> *If quiet never stays,*
> *movement increases and increases,*
> *Speculating too much is wasteful,*
> *and is not as good as protecting the flag.*
>
> — *Laozi*

This passage from Laozi's treatise, *Dao De Jing*, discusses the idea that there is no loving and compassionate god which oversees the universe. Laozi says that anyone who has true wisdom will also comport themselves as the world does. Rather than telling all people lies about the great compassion of the heavens, he will simply work to protect the people of his country.

The key idea here is that if we talk too much about esoteric things, it will cause people around us to react, either in belief or disbelief, and will begin to cause negative things to occur in society. People will lose their unknowing nature and become perverted by superstitious beliefs.

Just like all religious practice, Daoism changed after the time of Laozi, and many Daoist beliefs still hold elements of the Zhou dynasty religious practice as key elements of their religious practice.

Laozi did have one thing in common with the Zhou rulers, though – he believed that all things are unified by one great unchanging constant. The constant of Laozi is the *dao*.

Dao was later characterized in the Qing dynasty book, *Xing Ming Qui Zhi*, as being ineffable but brought together by *qi*.

More specifically, in the document *Da Dao Shuo, or "Speaking of the Great Dao,"* it is said:

"The Buddha classic has five thousand forty eight passages, and yet speaking it is not as good as understanding its structures... The Dao De Jing has five thousand important words, but speaking it is not as good as following its method fully. Only one thing can be said with sureness, and that is the word qi"

This word, *qi,* is what the Daoists believed to be the key to understanding all of the mysteries of creation. They believed the human body and the universe were made of the same energy and that if people learned to harness and control it, they would meld with the universe and become immortal.

Because the path of *qi* in the universe follows the *zhou tian,* "the heavenly orbit cycle" previously mentioned, it means that the body also does. The orbit of the universe is called *da zhou tian,* or "great heavenly orbit." The orbit of the body is called *xiao zhou tian,* or "small heavenly orbit."

They follow the same great path of energy which moves accordingly through the elixir field (*dantian*) to all places. The energy moving in the elixir field gradually strengthens it and causes people to be able to return to the elixir of the universe and to improve their situation by not only working with their own energy, but actually experiencing the energy around them as their own, being able to develop and use it rather than spending of their own resources.

The practice of *xiao zhou tian* in Daoism is a preliminary way to get to a higher level. The core of the practice revolves around using the mind to cause the *qi* to move up the body through the three gates of the back (*san guan*, mentioned earlier), up to the upper *dantian* of the head, and gradually back to the middle *dantian* of the chest, and finally to the lower *dantian* in the belly. This cycle can be repeated as often as required and can take anywhere from five minutes to one hour to complete.

Accomplished meditators will to some extent eventually abandon *xiao zhou tian* practice because, when they meditate, the energy will simply move to all places in their body—but this kind of practice is a very good way to establish a basic connective circuit in the body that the *qi* can follow.

Again, it should be stated that the method of making the energy move up the spine is simply to place the mind in the abdomen for long enough that it causes the feeling to naturally move on its own.

Once it has cleared the back and is in the head, the emphasis should only be placed on feeling the energy and on lightly breathing. When it feels like the energy has been there for long enough and is ready to move, then you can bring it back to the chest area—slowly opening and closing it with the breathing. Once the chest area feels relaxed and the energy is ready to move again, simply allow the energy to move to the lower *dantian*.

When you finish the meditation, you can just put the mind back in the lower *dantian* and let it rest there—or you can place the mind on the whole body and gradually open your eyes.

When you stand up from meditating, you should take care to do it slowly and with consciousness. This principle should also be applied to waking up in the morning or at night. Many people have accidents when they get up too fast. This is partly due to the fact that during sleep, all the blood in the body has moved to the head in order to protect the brain. When we wake up, if we move too fast, the blood will not have had enough time to circulate in the body – so if we stand up too quickly, it is easy to fall right over.

WAKE UP ELIXIR PRACTICE:

- ❖ When you get up each morning, you can do the following exercise to ease yourself into the day:

- ❖ Lie flat on your back in bed.

- ❖ Move your mind and breath to the lower *dantian* area of the abdomen.

- ❖ Feel the breathing slowly moving in and out, expanding and deflating naturally.

- ❖ Keep your mind there for a few minutes, and then place the mind into the legs and feet.

- ❖ Focus on softening the muscles in the legs, hips, waist and stomach, around the ribs, chest, shoulders, neck and face.

- ❖ Lie motionless for a few moments.

- ❖ Gradually stir your body by simply moving a few fingers, toes, hand, arm, or whatever part feels stiff and like it needs movement.

- ❖ Do this with all your appendages.

- ❖ Roll your head slightly from left to right, stopping in the middle each time for one full, relaxing breath.

- ❖ Rub the hands together and imagine you are using them to wash your face.

- ❖ Rub them together again and put them over your eyes for a few moments (this will help cure "sleepy eyes" in the morning).

- ❖ Slowly sit up in bed and give yourself a massage from the crown point of the head, the forehead and face, down to the chest, upper back, kidneys, abdomen, waist, hips, legs, knees, and down the calves to the feet.

- ❖ Dangle your legs over the edge of the bed and sit quietly there, feeling your breath coming and leaving for a few minutes.

❖ Put one foot and then the other on the floor – feel the floor with your feet and gradually adjust to the temperature.

❖ Gradually slip out of bed and stand up.

❖ Take a moment to gain your bearings while standing in silence.

❖ Have two small cups of water, drinking each sip deliberately and with an attention to the water softly moving down your throat to your belly.

❖ Go to the washroom and wash your face, brush your teeth, shower, and use the lavatory (in whichever order you like).

❖ Eat a square meal, and get your day started!

The essential practice of small heavenly orbit is to open up the torso to the feeling of moving energy. Gradually it will become possible to abandon the concept of *xiao zhou tian* and simply feel the energy as it moves naturally in the body. This may take from one year to a decade to perform correctly.

There will often be times when the energy feels blocked in the body. These blocks are almost always emotionally related. In fact, the only times when *qi* doesn't flow smoothly in the body is when the mind and breathing become fixed and can't move freely on their own.

The big goal of this and many other types of practice are to allow the mind, breath, and energy to freely circulate in harmony with each other.

As with all practices in Daoism, to do this correctly, you must focus on quiet and calm. You must also learn to slow down the thoughts and protect the empty and chaotic feeling in the lower *dantian*.

This will cause the *qi* to rise by itself—and then, once it rises to the head, you can control it by allowing it to open and close with the breath until it is ready to move again.

CHAPTER 4:

YIN AND YANG – ACTIVE AND PASSIVE FIRE

A big concept in Daoism is that of *yin* and *yang*. *Yin* is a female and passive type of energy in the universe. *Yang* is the active, male energy that permeates all things. Practicing *yin* and *yang* in alchemy meditation is considered to be related to two different types of fire: passive and active.

The term "fire" means the intensity with which one focuses the mind. The mind may be used to direct different levels of intent to the body and, as such, may cultivate energy at different levels of intensity.

Active and passive fire are conceptualized as being the best way to control the level of *qi* flowing in the body.

Essentially, the *qi* of the body has a tendency to go in one of two directions when we practice. It naturally slows down, and we become sleepy and confused, or else the *qi* becomes too excited, or too "hot."

This type of *qi*, while very effective in cycling energy, can be quite destructive, as the intensity of the mind may cause damage to the nervous system and allow the thoughts to become too hot.

People who practice extreme styles of yoga, qi gong, or meditation sometime experience a type of "energy burnout." This is because they practice with too much intent and don't know how to turn down the heat enough to get the full benefit of the practice without injuring themselves.

Over-reliance on passivity in energy practice is a hallmark of people who prefer to rest and relax, tend toward heavy eating, sleep unusually long hours, or are overweight.

Energetic extremity tends to occur in "over-achievers" and high-energy people. Often sports players will trend toward energetic exhaustion, and people with obsessive personalities often put too much reliance on an "active" mental state.

Using the concept of *yin* and *yang* to balance the energy in the body is not only useful in meditation, it can also be used as a life principle.

If you are a very active person, it may be a good idea to force yourself to slow down a few times a day and quite literally take time to breathe.

If you are a lethargic person, it is good to stir every once in a while and make sure to walk around, shaking off any kinks or tight muscles.

The active fire and passive fire practice work like this in meditation:

At the start of a meditation practice, it is normal to start in a somewhat neutral state—this state is the time when you are just feeling the breath moving in and out of the body.

As you begin to direct your mind to the lower *dantian*, you may wish to focus the mind there—as if shining a flashlight on the area. Gradually as your attention fixes, it will cause the energy feeling to begin to become apparent. This is often accompanied by a warm feeling in the *dantian*—but can also be similar to the feeling of wind blowing in the body.

Once the energy rises naturally up the spine to the head, you can rest your mind in the center of the head.

At this time, you can turn the heat down and simply focus on passively resting your attention on the breath and the feeling in and around the head.

If you start to feel sleepy, begin to focus the mind toward the third eye area on the front of the forehead and try to feel as though you are opening and closing the breath in that area.

Once the energy begins to move again, you can let it slowly move to the chest, and once all of the awareness arrives there, you may wish to slow down the mind a bit and focus on the feeling of the breath in the chest—start to relax the muscles behind the ribs and create a settling feeling.

It is usually good to stay soft when breathing in the chest because the chest area is associated with the heart and the emotions. If your chest is too active energetically, you may become overly excited and encounter emotional problems after practice. It is best to keep the mind focused on the passive fire stage at this point.

Once the *qi* moves to the lower *dantian*, it is best to let the energy settle completely before focusing the mind on activity again. Once you are totally relaxed, it is time to start moving the mind downward again in order to make the *qi* boil and move back up the body.

Keep in mind that both active and passive fire are subsets of each other—active fire being a true representation of *yang*—a male energy with a small dot of the female contained within it.

Passive fire is true *yin*—the female contained within the male – so the level of intensity you use in practice should never be completely masculine or completely feminine. This will allow you to gradually feel what level of intensity you need to apply to remain energetically balanced during and after practice.

CHAPTER 5

100 DAY FOUNDATION TRAINING

It is popularly believed in Daoism that, from the time of undertaking daily training, it will take nine years in total to achieve a high level of practice. This practice follows the principle that the body must first be allowed to repair itself and then begin to make progress toward developing a powerful and dynamic internal energy and spirit.

The most basic method of beginning this training is contained in the book, *Da Cheng Jie Yao*, or "The Great Success Shortcut Method," which is a Daoist classic written during the Ming/Qing era, around 400 years ago. *Da Cheng Jie Yao* was written for normal people who wanted to undertake Daoist training in order to help them live longer and become happier. The book is written in 24 sections, the first of which is called, "changing to emptiness and hiding in hibernation in the *qi xue*."

The term *qi xue* refers to an acupuncture point below the lower *dantian* (the area inside and around the lower abdomen), and literally means "energy cave" or "breath cave." It is considered as the very lowest part of the abdomen before the stomach area ends and the reproductive system begins. This area is associated with *xing*, or the sexual essence of the genitals, and the *ming* life essence of the kidneys. In Chinese medicine, this area is known as the *ming men*, or "life gate (see pg. 22 for location reference)."

Daoist people think that if the mind is placed in the *qi* cave, the meditator will gradually forget their thoughts, and their intention will gradually settle in the abdomen. This period can be treated as a type of hibernation exercise.

The idea of hibernation is also similar to the practice of developing an "energetic embryo" which is discussed in the following passage from the *Jade Emperor's Embryonic-breathing Classic*:

"The embryo congeals as the breath enters the centre— the energy develops as the embryo rests in the centre." The concept at play is that if one is able to relax the abdomen and fuse the breathing and intention together there, it will gradually cause certain feelings to develop. One such feeling is the area around the abdomen begins to heat up slightly, and, eventually, the area feels alive."

Daoists believe that this "alive" feeling is actually the creation of an energy embryo in the belly, and this embryo is the beginning level of Daoist energetic practice. In the

Da Cheng Jie Yao it is suggested that this practice must be undertaken for at least 100 days. This idea is summed up in the following passage:

> **"In order to enter the hibernation practice, you must use the mind to stir the essence (jing), and awaken the essence to refine it into energy (qi)."**

This brings us back to the concept of *jing, qi,* and *shen*—the three treasures of Daoism. At this stage of training, the most basic concept is that we must make our minds calm and place our spirit (*shen*) into the lower abdomen in order to begin cultivating the essence (*jing*).

This process should be treated in a very calm way. The thoughts must be forgotten, and the mind must go into the *wuwei* or "non-action" state. The idea at play is that the mind should be allowed to rest and achieve a state of balance. The reason why this training is considered like hibernation is that when the mind rests in the abdomen, it may take a long time to wake up the energy there. During this time, the meditator will gain the benefit of slowing down the thoughts, relaxing the body, naturally fixing the posture, and regulating the breathing. Eventually, the energy will begin to move on its own. *The mind in no way moves the energy.* Instead, the energy should just naturally emerge.

The key to the 100 day hibernation phase is not to actively begin moving the energy, but instead to set up the

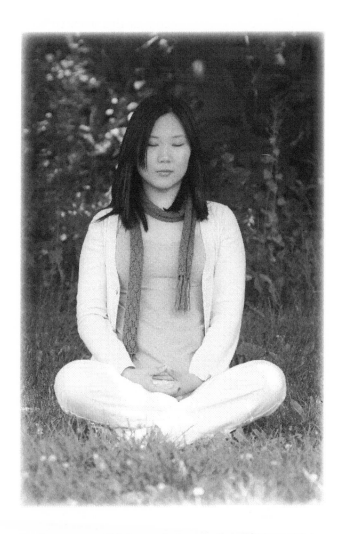

Meditation posture: This is a typical meditation posture which is easy for beginners. Simply sit down, cross the legs, lightly close the eyes, and cup the hands together at the waist. For those with limited mobility, it is also possible to adapt this posture to sitting upright in a chair, simply retain the posture but let the legs naturally extend to the floor.

basic requirements for the energy body to open up and begin developing.

The phrase "100 days" is also not exact. This type of practice could take as few as a couple of weeks and all the way up to one year to establish. Every person is different, and each person has their own level of ability to feel energy. This practice is more about feeling than doing, so you should simply follow the feeling, and if the energy begins to move upward, just allow it to happen. If the energy rises to the head, simply let it rest there until it naturally moves downward to the chest and then returns to the abdomen.

If the energy does not move, simply keep the mind in the *qi* cave until you begin to gain some results from the practice.

The breathing during this time should be slow, calm, and natural. The breath should always feel as though it is moving downward. The abdomen is allowed to slightly inflate on the in-breath, and slightly deflate on the out-breath. The mind should always move toward the *qi* cave and earth.

This practice can be done seated, standing, or lying down, cross legged, or in a chair. The posture of the body should feel natural and not forced. The mouth should be closed with the teeth touching lightly and the tongue resting with its tip to the roof of the mouth. During the very first stages of training, you can just sit back in a comfortable chair and feel the breath entering and leaving your body.

The Daoist master Hu Haiya told my teacher, Yang Hai, "My teacher advised me to begin meditation by sitting back, relaxing, and feeling the breath." As such, this practice should be comfortable and natural. It can produce many different types of results but should never become uncomfortable, overly energetic, or forced.

During this practice you may feel any number of things, including:

❖ The breath beginning to slow down.

❖ The mind becoming quiet and calm.

❖ The opening and closing of the diaphragm and belly during breathing.

❖ The mind settling in the centre of the body.

❖ Sensations of mild heat or tingling around the lower abdomen.

❖ A feeling of unclarity or a mixing of emotions which has no concrete definition.

❖ A "spark" or subtle beginning of energetic action in the abdomen.

❖ You may see light or colours behind the eyes.

❖ A feeling of the posture straightening and becoming more comfortable.

❖ Dramatic relaxation of the muscles of the torso.

❖ Feelings of deep comfort and happiness.

❖ A movement which runs upward along the inside of the back and up to the head.

❖ A sudden feeling of consciousness or energy in the entire body.

❖ Opening and clarifying sensations in the head, skull, and brain.

❖ Similar feelings in the chest, heart, and lungs.

❖ Feelings of deep peace and insight.

❖ Changes in the way that you perceive reality.

❖ New ideas or feelings about life.

❖ A sense of kindness and connection to the universe.

All of these sensations are good and mean that your practice is moving in the correct direction.

The main point is that you should not become excited during practice and should maintain a sense of calm detachment.

If you suddenly become afraid, or have difficulty facing emotions during practice, the best things to do is just quietly observe the emotions coming and going - as long as your thought process does not begin to "grab" the feelings which arise. The feelings will naturally pass after a few moments.

The goal of this level of practice is to begin clarifying the energy and mind in order to allow the spirit to begin to reside in the body. Unlike Descartes, the Daoists believe that one's spirit is not separate from one's body, and so the body and spirit must be cultivated together and allowed to become healthy at the same time.

CHAPTER 6:

XUAN MEN – MYSTERY GATE

Daoists use the idea of "emptiness" to help them practice understanding the world at large.

Laozi frequently mentions emptiness in passages such as the following one translated from the *Mawangdui Dao De Jing* manuscript, the oldest existing manuscript of the *Dao De Jing*:

"If you are long without desire, you may see the subtlety (of the dao); always with desire, there is only shouting! These two move together but are named differently in the same belly. Its meaning is mystery, the mystery of the dark, and the door to that which is invisible."

This passage means that people who wish to see the *dao* must always hold themselves without earthly desires. If they always desire for material things, their thoughts will be violent and forever seem like the sound of shouting. Laozi says that even though these ideas look different, they emerge from the same source (the *dao*), and that if we want to understand, we have to go beyond what is obvious. *It is important to research emptiness in order to see beyond what is available to our five senses.*

The most important concept here is that of *xuan*. In ancient Chinese *xuan* means "darkness" or "blackness," but Laozi uses it to discuss the principle of "mystery." Mystery is that which is not well known, but has some sense of possibility. Although something is not known to us, it does not mean that it does not exist. Our ability to peer into the unknown and take benefit from it is one of the best ways to improve life.

The modern consciousness teacher, Peter Ralston, often says that he never learned anything he already knew. And so when the *Dao De Jing* discusses *xuan*, it can be interpreted as being somewhere between mystery, darkness, and not knowing.

Not knowing is an attitude which can be held during meditation practice in order to stop the mind from making the assumption of understanding reality. If one already assumes they have understood reality, then the job of study is already over as there is nothing new to learn. When people learn to at least give up some of their own understanding, they effectively create room to add new details to their current understanding of reality.

Observing not knowing is as simple as sitting in silence and abandoning the desire to use verbal thought to communicate with oneself. It can also be carried in many other types of practice, some of which we will discuss a bit later.

Daoists also talk about a type of practice known as *xuan men*, which, in Daoism, is somewhat like a black belt in the martial arts. It is the gate between the beginner level of practice and a higher level of insight and ability within the framework of meditation.

In fact, *xuan men* means "mystery gate." This phase of Daoism is not clear, as many different groups have interpreted the principle differently. It can mean the practitioner has become enlightened, or it can simply infer that one's practice has emerged from the state of non-action to the state of action without action.

This type of ability is not a beginner level skill in Daoism, but it is important to know what it is, so that if encountered, it can be understood, and the mind of the practitioner will not become chaotic.

One of the first major interpretations of *xuan men* is from the book, *Wu Zhen Pian* or "Understanding Reality." It says that when people reach the *xuan men* level of practice, they may meditate for a very long time, but when they emerge from meditation, it will seem as if they have only practised for a few minutes. In fact, several hours may have already gone by.

This phase of practice essentially means that the nervous system has been allowed to rest completely, and the mind has truly let go and stopped holding onto arbitrary thoughts.

This does not mean that you should fall asleep when you practice, or that you should lose consciousness in any way. In fact, you should become increasingly aware of the world within and without, but at the time of entering the mystery gate stage, it may seem as if the time you spent in practice was actually much shorter than it really was.

Mystery gate is not a term which is mutually agreed on across the board in Daoism. It can also be a part of practice which occurs during individual practice sessions. So, in effect, the mystery gate is the result of successful meditation practice. It is the time at which the practice goes from the consciously controlled "post-natal state," to the unconsciously controlled "pre-natal state."

This means that the practice stops being something which the "intention" controls and becomes something that regulates itself automatically, without the activation of intent. This phase is comparable to the states of *wu wei* and *wei wu wei*, where the mind gradually begins to acclimatize to total silence and relaxation.

Both of these views of *xuan men* are correct, and it can be considered something which is either entered after a long period of practice and is the gate to a higher stage of more refined practice, or as something which is frequently attained in order to regulate the practice beyond the mere use of intention to drive the function of energy movement.

A GREATER DISCUSSION OF WU WEI

At the start of the book, we briefly touched on the subject of *wu wei* or non-action. This principle is one of the greatest keys to Daoist practice.

The non-action state is essentially the phase of meditation during which the mind has more or less relaxed completely. It is also the phase where there is no attachment to individual thoughts which may occur. Although the mind is always processing information, when we enter deep meditation we can stop the mind from taking in new visual and verbal stimulation. Consider the difference between going from a room with loud music and people dancing, and then all of a sudden being placed into a quiet and secluded garden. This is somewhat akin to the experience of calming the mind through meditation. *Wu wei* is one of the results of this event.

Essentially, when we quiet the mind fully, it will stop actively processing and thinking about new information for long enough that the psyche can begin to relax itself. This is somewhat akin to charging a battery, but instead of filling the battery with electricity, we are instead charging our consciousness. When the mind reaches a certain level of non-action, it will gradually work to relax the muscles, slow the breathing, and calm the nerves.

Many beginner meditators mistake the complete calming of the nervous system for enlightenment itself but, in fact, the levels of calm and quietude achieved during this state are just an indication that the mind has reached the non-action phase of meditation.

Beyond w*u wei* is another concept called *wei wu wei*, which means "action without action."

This state comes when the mind has been calmed for a long time and the meditation begins to deeply heal the already relaxed nervous system. This state is related to the mystery gate in that it is the phase in which people forget themselves and lose track of time. This is not to say that the mind becomes unconscious, just that it begins to lose its sense of value-based judgement.

At this time it is possible to not think, not worry, and not do anything which requires the input of the active mind of day-to-day life. This is also the point at which the energy of the body will wake up to its fullest potential and move on its own. It is also the point at which the body will become truly natural and accord itself with the world as opposed to attempting to force the world to accord with it. In a sense, *wei wu wei* could be phrased in English as "going with the flow."

The value of these two states is in the deep sense of rest and relaxation they create.

It is very rare for people to relax completely, and sleep is generally the only time the nervous system is given to not act and simply be. If we are able to spend even half an hour every day without thinking about our next activity, we may actually begin to undertake the real healing of our bodies and minds that sleep cannot accomplish by itself.

SOCIETY AND WU WEI

It seems as if television, computers, advertising, and media of all kinds have overtaken our lives, and because we are always subject to ever greater bombardment of the senses, many people are undergoing a serious "media fatigue." Most people are unaware the level to which media control us, but they do know that they are exhausted.

Since the 1970s, children have grown up in ever greater states of technological dependence.

It used to be possible for children in towns and cities to take a walk in nature and to learn from the world around them. Now the majority of learning takes place behind a computer screen. Not only are computers bad for physical posture, they also constantly attack our eyes and brains with excessive light, images, and neural messages which assault our subconscious and pervert our thinking.

A common problem among youth today is the ever growing trend to withdraw from the company of others and to be insulated in the fantasy world of the internet. This is leading to a whole multitude of social issues such as dependency, cyber bullying, violence against peers and families, and so on.

A key lesson which parents can give their children is how to take "time out" and evaluate their situation at large. The way parents do this and the way their children do will be different, but both can accord to the *wu wei* principle.

If adults wish to have some true quiet time for reflection, they may simply sit quietly in meditation with the mind following the breath. This will eventually lead to quiet and relaxation of the nerves which are all too often overwhelmed by outside information.

Children are not well suited to silent meditation, so they may be taught non-action through activities which force them to focus only on one task. Excellent physical pursuits such as sports, the martial arts, and physical exercise are one important route to getting the mind focused and becoming calmer. Other activities like art, music, or even various kinds of high-involvement play time can also cause the minds of children to enter a place of rest and focus.

This also makes it easier to introduce more profound concepts such as ethics and the value of hard work. Later on, many people who study hobbies seriously as a child can go on to achieving insight that is greater than those who were simply allowed to idle in front of a screen while being constantly attacked by information and the sickness of a "plug in" addicted society.

Because *wu wei* is a passive practice, it is not something which can be forced; it simply needs to occur as a natural part of meditation. Simply sit down in a comfortable chair, relax the body, breathe to the center, close the eyes, and calm the mind. Eventually the body and mind will naturally incline toward the non-action state. The great thing about *wu wei* is that you can stay that way however long you wish and only gain benefit from it. Make sure you don't fall asleep though!

CHAPTER 7

XIAN TIAN, HOU TIAN -
BEFORE AND AFTER BIRTH

Daoism always views the world through the lens of *yin* and *yang*, so it is no surprise there are many different ways by which to speak of the occurrence of positive and negative energy in the universe.

The idea of positive and negative is not that one energy is better than the other, but instead, that just like a battery, all things have opposing charges that cause them to come to life. Without one, it would not be possible to have the other.

One of the most important concepts in Daoist cultivation is *xian tian, hou tian* which roughly means "before birth" and "after birth." These two occurrences can be characterized as being similar to a time when something has not yet occurred but is in the first stages of fruition, and then the stage when something has already developed and is concrete. Like an embryo which has yet to develop completely into a fetus, but is already mid-way through the first development stages of life, the *xian tian*, or "pre-heaven" phase, is the time when the most development is happening. It is also an unclear time, because there is no outside experience by which to measure it. An embryo does not know it is an embryo, nor can anyone see the very first stages of a seedling as it is germinating in grassy soil. This phase is the one that Daoists seek to emulate during meditation on non-action.

Hou tian, or the "after birth" phase of practice, is every kind of external sensation that occurs during meditation. This means that the initial use of the mind to wake up the *jing* and *qi* is considered within Daoism to be a kind of required physical input to begin moving toward the phase of merging with nature and becoming like an embryo during practice – or, more clearly, to establish the type of practice in which energy moves by itself and the body goes into a state of subconscious healing and renewal. Just like a child in the womb is in constant development with very little external input aside from the general heath of the pregnant mother, the *xian tian* phase of Daoism is the phase in which the universe nurtures the individual in meditation.

Xian tian has two types of occurrence. Just like the mystery gate, the pre-heaven phase of Daoism can be applied both to daily practice and to the long term. In daily practice, *xian tian* simply means that the person meditating should forget the self and meditate not as an ego, but rather use their entire being to enter a deep state of peace and rest.

In the long term, the pre-birth state is considered to be "changing old into young." It is a lifelong process of developing an ever greater level of physical and emotional health and vitality.

Hou tian, or "post-birth," also always follows two paths. The first is that the body must be maintained through proper diet and exercise as well as control of sleep cycles, sexual function, social relationships, etc. The second phase is the life-long process by which the exterior body is nourished by the *qi* that is taken in through breathing, the sun, and diet. This energy helps to protect the *jing*, or "pre-natal" energy in the abdomen. So, in effect, the *hou tian* protects the *xian tian*.

Pre-birth and post-birth are akin to the idea of non-action and action without action. They also have a relationship with the mystery gate in that the mystery gate is the barrier between pre- and post-birth practice. Essentially, practice will always be relegated to the post-birth phase until the practitioner can pass through the gate of *shen ming* or the "unclarity" state. Once in meditation for a long enough time, the "true mind," or *zhen yi,* will begin to act on its own and does not need instructions from the intention mind. The true mind simply regulates the body as required and will eventually pass through the *shen ming* state and into a state of clarity and emotional non-attachment.

This phase of practice is truly beautiful and can be achieved for the first time within a few months of beginning meditation but will often disappear and take a very long time to regain. Once it is regained, the state will be more permanent and easier to attain.

Stick with the practice and even if it doesn't seem like you have made much progress, keep going, and eventually you will begin to see what the true practice of pre- and post-birth, non-action and action without action, and the mystery gate are.

Although this practice takes many years, the benefits of the practice can be seen right from the outset. The mind may become calmer, and you may begin to feel able to tackle and resolve problems in your life. The true benefit of Daoism is cultivation of a better life. Keep that in mind as you practice and make progress!

CHAPTER 8:

SAYINGS OF LAOZI

Although Daoist meditation existed before the time of Laozi (early records of meditation and *qigong* can be found in cave paintings from Mongolia tracing back to the time before the Three Sovereigns and Five Emperors—First Dynasty of China, over 5000 years ago), Laozi was the first person to put the philosophy of Daoism into a clear and concise single written document.

The *Dao De Jing* is a collection of 82 chapters on the subject of how to establish a relationship with the nature of reality in all aspects of life.

Laozi's principle is that although it may not be possible to understand everything in the universe, it is possible to understand the fundamental principles which govern the universe. Laozi believed that these principles were all unified by their common relationship with emptiness and that they could be discovered by observing quiet.

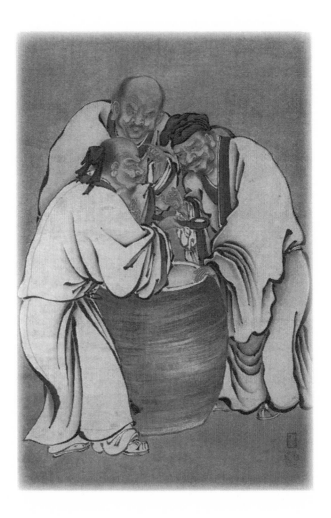

The vinegar tasters: This image of Laozi, Confucius, and the Buddha illustrates how Chinese people view the three tracks of spiritual life (Daoism, Confucianism, and Buddhism). Although Buddha and Confucius are both making pained faces while drinking vinegar, Laozi is laughing, since for him, it is a new experience. Daoists view the world as positive and every experience as having potential benefit.

If we use the universe as a model for the *dao*, then we can use quiet reflection as a model of the d*e*, or the way of observing the universe. Laozi believed people ought not to clutter their minds with useless thought and that, in communications, they should always remain neutral and not say more than needed.

The *Dao De Jing* is a very complex book, but it always returns to one fundamental principle, which is that of remaining calm, quiet, and observing things as they occur, rather than attaching value judgements to them before they happen.

As such, there are many pearls of wisdom which are applicable to meditation contained within Laozi's book. Some people even view the *Dao De Jing* as fundamentally being a work on the practice of meditation, and that the *de* is the true method of using the mind to cultivate the *dao* within oneself.

Daoist scholars call this type of practice *dao de nei guan,* or "the way of observing the *dao* through inner reflection."

Following are some statements of Laozi which are useful to improve the practice of meditation. Each passage will be accompanied by an explanatory paragraph, to help get you started on your practice.

Still the heart,
Fill the belly,
Soften the will,
Strengthen the bones.

This passage is about how to set up the basic criteria of meditation. It is from Chapter Three of the *Dao De Jing* and is commonly considered to mean that when people meditate, they should calm the emotional mind. In this case, the emotional mind is signified by the heart. In Chinese philosophy, the emotions are considered to come from the heart, which is no surprise, as most positive and negative feelings emanate and move out from the chest area. So when Laozi says to still the heart, he means both that true meditation requires a quiet mind and also balanced emotions. It is not possible to achieve true meditation until the mind is calm and the emotions and thoughts stop running wild.

Next, he says to fill the belly. This means that when we breathe, it is important to allow the breath to fully settle into the abdominal area and *dantian*. This means that the breath can't be carried in the chest; it must sink the whole way to the base of the spine. This will naturally cause the posture to begin straightening, and the mind to become calm.

Softening the will means that we must stop ourselves from feeling as though we are "working." Daoist meditation practice is based on the concept of water flowing freely from place to place, so when we meditate, we must not be overly focused on any specific objective - simply breathe, relax, remain calm, and let the mind move naturally of its own accord.

Strengthening the bones is both a practice and a result of meditation. The practice of strengthening the bones simply means that it is important to sit in a stable posture and remain unmoving. It also means that you are required to focus on the interior of the body rather than the outside. The bones represent the core of the body, so strengthening the bones is another way to say that meditators should not focus too much on the outside of the body and mind.

The result of this practice taken as a whole is that it strengthens the inner resolve of the practitioner and can lead to positive changes in lifestyle which come from within. Strengthening the bones, in effect, means that when we meditate, we are trying to make the inner workings of our beings stronger.

Much like running and push-ups make the muscles strong, Daoists thought it was important to make the energy strong, the breath move freely, and to create a sense of "life" emerge from the centre of their beings and envelop them in calm and happiness.

Some sayings of Laozi are as short as a few characters – such as the concept of *duo yan qiong*: "Talking too much is a poor choice," and *Shou Zhong*: "protecting the centre"

—but others need to be used in reference to whole chapters of the book.

Let's have a look at Chapter Four of the *Dao De Jing*:

> *The way is empty/turbid*
> *and it cannot be used completely.*
> *It is vastly deep,*
> *and is the ancestor of all beings.*
> *(The way)*
> *blunts sharpness,*
> *relieves confusion,*
> *comes together with the light,*
> *and joins with the dust.*
> *It is completely clear in its existence.*
> *I don't know whose son it is.*
> *It seems to have existed even before god.*

The key points of this passage are the emphasis on going from being unclear and empty in the non-action state, to gradually moving the true mind into the essence (*jing*). In this case, "the ancestor of all beings" is the *jing* energy, which arises simply as a bi-product of conception.

The next part of the instruction is about how to hold the mind during meditation. We should remove the edges from our perception. This means that we should avoid allowing the practice to take on a defined shape, but rather to stay in the chaotic state. The natural bi-product of this will be to cut away confused thoughts and allow us to attain the *ming*, or "brightness" state. At the same time, we also must remember to rest in non-action - which means we have to be content to settle in the dust of obscurity during practice. Even if we want to get up and move around, it is very important to remain still and formless. This will naturally result in pure clarity of the consciousness and, in the opinion of Laozi, reveal the state of emptiness that existed even before the creation of the universe.

The whole *Dao De Jing* can be read as a great code for meditation, but one of the biggest problems to contemporary readers is that classical Chinese is obscure and can take on many different meanings and contexts. The good news is that anyone who has read this book up to this point will be able to begin taking instructions directly from the source. You can simply get any copy of *Dao De Jing* (there are many translations available), and begin to research for yourself. Keep in mind that the central message of Laozi never changes. He believed in peace and non-contention among people.

He also believed in conservation and not doing more than needed. If you take this as method of practice, you will be less likely to make mistakes along the way.

CHAPTER 9:

YIN AND YANG IN DAOIST MEDITATION PRACTICE

One of the biggest intellectual aspects associated with Daoism is the theory of *yin* and *yang*.

Although *yin* and *yang*—as the principle of male and female, or positive- and negative-charged energy in the universe—predates Daoism, it is one of the standards which sets Daoism apart from other religious practices. Instead of looking at the *yang*, or positive, as good and *yin*, or negative, as evil, Daoism looks at both as required parts of the other. *Yin* always eventually turns into *yang* as *yang* turns to *yin*.

Laozi said:

"Consider how empty and full exist in each other, difficulty and ease change into each other, long and short are elements of each other, top and bottom rest on each other, sound and noise blend together, back and front chase each other."

This is the basic Daoist idea of how *yin* and *yang* work in the world. Everything that is *yang* is supported by *yin*, and everything that is *yin* is brought to life by *yang*. This has the ultimate result of *yin* and *yang* being the manifestation which all sentient beings may observe as the movement and change of nature.

By now, it should be evident that the majority of practices in this book are about how to properly balance *yin* and *yang* in meditation in order to make the energy of the body more abundant and the mind more peaceful.

Daoism as a practice is fundamentally rooted in creating something from nothing – or more exactly, the focus on the soft and feminine in order to create the strong and dynamic.

Daoism views the ultimate outcome of concentration on the *yin* aspect of our being as being the birth and growth of the dynamic *yang* nature which we are trying to become.

This is not to say that *yin* means non-existence or that *yang* means a full abundance of life.

Although we were not fully sentient in the womb, we still existed and fed on the *yin* energy of our mothers. Just as we did that, we also grew and developed, which is the exact analogy that Daoists use to describe the process of elixir meditation. Simply by calming ourselves and allowing non-action, we allow ourselves to gain energy and eventually become much more active than we previously imagined possible.

This is the true movement of yin and yang in Daoism.

BASIC MEDITATION PRACTICE OF DAOIST ELIXIR ALCHEMY

- ❖ Sit upright on the edge of a chair.

- ❖ Fold your hands at your waist, or put your hands on your knees palm down.

- ❖ Close your eyes and relax your mind while focusing on the feeling of your breaths moving slowly in and out.

- ❖ Begin to imagine the space around your entire body and gradually pull your attention inward and downward toward the belly button.

- ❖ Gradually move the mind deeper into the abdomen and downward into the *dantian* area just a few inches under the belly button.

- ❖ Simply let the mind rest there and breathe naturally.

- ❖ It is okay at this point if your breath becomes either shallow or deeper; simply remain relaxed with your mind focused on the core of your body.

- ❖ If the mind wanders, bring it back to the *dantian* as soon as you catch it.

- ❖ Once you are comfortable, continue moving the mind downward and toward the *qi xue* point between the dantian and genitals.

- ❖ Continue to breathe naturally and simply observe the phenomenon in the abdomen.

- ❖ Stay this way for a long time and do not attempt to make the energy move by doing anything other than restfully observing your breath.

- ❖ If the energy begins to move up the back, simply allow it to move naturally and by itself.

- ❖ If it moves up the front, put the mind back in the abdomen and don't let it rise. If it doesn't move, simply remain natural, with the mind on the *qi xue* point.

All people react differently to meditation, and everyone's body is different, so there is no sure way to tell how long it will take to create the energy sensation. For some people it can happen within days, for others in takes years. Even if the energy doesn't feels like it moves, simply focusing on the abdomen will naturally boil the *jing,* and the energy will circulate.

If you feel the energy very strongly, this is a good thing. Let the feeling move by itself and, when it arrives at the head, simply let it rest there. Continue breathing softly and begin to focus the attention on the energy feeling in the head.

At this point you should be aware of the balance of *yin* and *yang* in the body and whether or not you need to turn up the "heat" of the intention, or make it "cooler" by softening the focus of the mind. In either way, the mind should gradually begin to settle and become quiet.

Once it feels like the energy wants to move again, simply allow your mind to gradually settle in your chest. Follow the same instructions you used with your head, and simply breathe in and out naturally while adjusting the amount of intent you use as needed. The body should feel natural and not be forced into any specific posture. If the body bows a bit, simply let it work by itself. If the posture straightens, let it do so, but don't force it.

Once the energy needs to move again, simply direct it back to the *dantian*. If you want to end the meditation, settle the mind in the *dantian* and then focus on the whole body, breathing naturally, and then open the eyes and take a few minutes to acclimatize to the light and air in the room.

If you want to keep going, simply move the mind back down to the *qi xue* point and repeat the process.

You can do this as many times as you like and focus on the circulation for as long as you want, but usually people do this for between 15 minutes to one hour. More than that may make your body stiff, so you might want to stand up and move around a bit in breaks during long sessions.

Don't be overly focused on practice. If something is required of you somewhere else, you should be able to bring yourself back and take care of it. It is advisable, though, to avoid too much outside interference during practice. You should turn off the radio and your phone, and avoid meditating in loud places or places where there is a great deal of sensory input going on.

Meditation is best when it feels good and natural, so you ought not to have any mental disturbances or extreme feelings. If you feel uncomfortable when you meditate, simply bring yourself back into the room, and go for a walk outside.

You should always mix with people a few hours after meditating. This way you can observe how the practice interacts with your sense of well-being in the social realm. This is very important because sometimes we can be tricked into the romantic notion of becoming solitary and avoiding others in favour of developing our spirits.

Unless we are completely dedicated and willing to abandon our lives altogether, it is much better to use meditation as a tool for improving our lives both in the personal and social realm.

There is a saying that the monks with the greatest level of achievement are not in temples or caves, but instead are mixed in among normal people and living normal lives.

When you meditate, you should always attempt to stabilize yourself and improve your situation.

Focus on positivity and the feeling of kindness and righteousness. Share the happiness you achieve while meditating in your interactions with other people.

This type of generosity is the true root of spiritual practice and should be observed by all who are involved in meditation.

CHAPTER 10:

DOCUMENT REVIEW -
LU ZU BAI ZI BEI

Lu Dongbin's 100 character ancestor stone is one of the earliest defining works of Daoist meditation practice. Lu was born in the late Eight Century and was an important poet, scholar, and philosopher of the Tang dynasty.

Lu and his teacher Han Zhongli were seminal in creating the "golden elixir internal cultivation" school of Daoism, which was the first school to clearly emphasize meditation practice and enlightenment as the main purpose of Daoist cultivation.

There are many different poems associated with Lu Dongbin, but his "100 characters" is the most important because it gives a complete explanation of the effects of meditation and how to correctly practice in order to gain "internal medicine" and "climb the ladder to heaven." Below is a translation and explanation of Lu's poem, using other Daoist texts and ideas to cross reference and fill in the blanks.

The first several phrases have the longest explanations since they contain the key criteria of correct practice. The later phrases describe the overall effect of meditation and hint at some of the possible mental manifestations of correct practice.

To cultivate qi, forget to say "protect."

This phrase technically means that if a person desires to nurture the intrinsic energy of their being, they should not try to maintain the activity of the thinking mind during meditation.

The phrase "*yang qi*" has a literal meaning of cultivating and nurturing a type of energy which must be built-up rather than being inherently available like oxygen or intention. This *qi* differs from the more commonly used character which indicates "oxygen," "feeling," or "activity."

This *qi*, in fact, refers to the ability to use the mind to refine energy from an empty and silent source. It is a combination of the character "*wu*," meaning "empty" or "non-existing," and the character "*huo*," meaning "fire." Placing fire below an empty place, in this sense, refers to a process similar to boiling water, or more importantly in Chinese thought, smelting metal into a workable form.

Early Daoists were deeply interested in the process of alchemy and believed that certain metals when smelted could revert naturally to their original form after cooling. They believed that this process could be applied to the human body and allow people to become immortal, to discard the body, and live eternally in a purely spiritual realm.

This concept was originally used as a method by which to create an elixir to be taken internally in an attempt to cure mortality. These elixirs often proved to be fatal, and as such, were eventually fully replaced by the practice of meditation. Many meditation texts retained the elixir terminology in an effort to clarify how to process of meditation worked. The early Daoists believed that it was possible to use the mind to temper the sexual essence of the body into a type of golden elixir which could cause the spirit to awaken, lighten, and become immortal.

Lu Dongbin was an early proponent of this concept and argued that this internal elixir practice should replace the attempts to use refined metal as a spiritual medicine.

His language reflects the earlier external alchemy practice and begins to discuss how the same principle may be applied to the beneficial practice of meditation.

Wang yan shou, literally means "to forget to speak the word protect," but as with all documents emerging from the Daoist genre, it should not be taken literally.

Wang yan shou actually means that when we are concerned with developing energy in the body, we should assume a mental posture in which we do not attempt to hold on to verbal logic and thought. Rather, it is superior to forget one's sense of propriety and simply engage naturally in a state of pure, unfiltered consciousness. This also does not mean that it is desirable to stop thoughts from occurring, but rather to allow them to come and go freely, without interruption by the aspect of the mind which is concerned with attaching value to things.

Laozi famously said in the *Dao De Jing*:

"All the gold and the jade in the palace cannot be protected. To be rich, important, and arrogant is a punishment in itself. When your work is done, disappear and return to the way of heaven."

This assertion strongly supports Lu's idea of "*wang yan shou*," in that it suggests it is genuinely impossible to protect oneself from divisive behaviour if it comes from one's own mind. The suggestion to simply return to the way of heaven after all work is finished is another way to advise that we should not become attached to accomplishment. This is an extremely important concept in Lu's meditation method, and so he advises "to nurture the *qi*, one must forget to say protect."

This also fits nicely with Laozi's idea that:

Everyone in the world knows that beauty is beautiful.
This is already evil.
All know that good is good.
This is already not good.

Because it suggests that if we wish to truly be happy, and not damage our energy, we should avoid thinking in terms of absolutes. Instead of absolutes of good and bad, we should recognize all things as mixed. Imagine this to be like the difference between a black and white world and a world of colours. The mind must be made to accommodate the possibility of a world of subtle nuance rather than a world where all things are clear.

One of the first great lessons of meditation is that thoughts are temporary manifestations of the ego mind. Thoughts come and go as long as they are not clutched on to by the emotional mind.

Much opinion and belief is based on the desire for the mind not to be thrown into chaos.

"*Yang qi, wang yan shou*," is another way to say that if we do not attach too much significance to our thoughts, we will feel nourished and at peace.

Focus the heart on action without action.

The second phrase of the poem tells us to allow the body to settle into a state of non-doing and to be without motive.

The term *wu wei*, or "non-action" is Laozi's original concept of not forcing events to occur by one's will. This idea is the genuine hallmark of Daoism and is the concept of the entire practice.

In order to attain a high level of awareness, calm, and circulation of the breath and intrinsic energy, we must first void the mind of thought and desire. This non-action state can also be referred to as "non-motive" because one of the key concepts is that we should not hold judgement in our minds during the occurrence of this state. Typically, Daoist meditation practices are predicated upon first entering the non-action state and then, as the mind becomes still and silent, going beyond that into the *wei wu wei*, or "action without action" state.

Wei wu wei, at least in terms of meditation theory, is the time when all things that were previously at rest and calm become dynamic and alive. This idea is related to how the parasympathetic nervous system regulates the function of the body during sleep and healing. The goal of *jin dan* meditation is not to fall asleep but to mimic the level of rest and calm that is achieved in sleep and then go further by simply allowing the nervous and endocrine systems to function by themselves. When this is achieved, the body will begin to feel as though it is naturally filled with breath, energy, and sensation. Daoism refers to this state as entering into the mysterious gate.

At this time, the energy of the body is focused on softness and non-contention and according to Laozi...

To focus the breath completely on softness, one would become like a child.

This means that when we meditate, we should forget about the dirtiness and worry of the adult world, and simply revert to being flexible, soft, and natural just like a young child. Using non- action as our guide, we can gradually move into a deeper state where the body simply regulates itself without our conscious input.

So, according to Lu Dongbin, to "focus the heart on acting without action" is the way in which we may begin the act of cultivating energy in ourselves.

This phrase relates to the first phrase as a continuation of the idea that in order to cultivate energy, we must give up our ability to control the realm of our thoughts. Not only can we not protect ourselves at this time, but we must also abandon any motive for self-benefit during this time.

Laozi said:

The five colours make peoples' eyes blind,
the five sounds make peoples' ears deaf,
the five tastes make people's mouths unable to feel,
galloping hunting horses through the fields makes ones'
heart cold,
expensive and hard to obtain items stop one from being a
good person.
It is the sage who thinks with his belly instead of his eyes,
before he goes to grasp something better.

This is the moral heart of *Wu wei* and is the place in which the ideal of acting only based on need and not on want comes to the greatest prominence in Daoist philosophy.

One of the central tennets of all good meditation traditions is that the practitioner must abandon personal goals before they can become enlightened. Daoism holds that people wishing to cultivate themselves should not have to give up the good things in life like nice food, social activity, and sex, but instead should regulate them in such a way that they do not become addicted.

One of the goals of entering the non-action state is to show us how our desires manipulate us.

When we are completely silent and without thought of our own benefit, it becomes very clear that the world of earthly desire is false, without meaning, and not as good as simply existing in calm and awareness.

Directing the heart to non-action is the real first step of meditation in Lu Dongbin's *Jin Dan* school.

Move quietly, know the ancestral progenitor.

This phrase of the poem is extremely difficult to understand and very easy to misinterpret.

The phrase "*Dong jing,*" has the actual meaning of *wei wu wei*, or "acting without action," as its central meaning. "*Dong*" means "to move" and "*Jing*" means quiet, so together it indicates a type of movement occurring in a non-active place.

The key here is that there is a continuation of the previously discussed state of non-action which occurs after complete quiet and calm have been achieved. This stage is the time in Chinese cosmology before things are generated. It is called "*yin yun*" and is a kind of primordial event where living beings are generated from complete stillness. Lu Dongbin has inserted this idea into the phrase "*Dong Jing*," in order to help us understand the correct frame of mind to adopt in deep meditation. Although the mind becomes quiet and still, it will eventually begin to generate a feeling that moves through the whole body.

Huo Yuanji refers to this feeling in his book *Dao De Jing Chan Wei*, as *yi jue*, or "single inspiration." Inspiration is not the exact word to describe this event, but this moment of shifting into action without action is similar to a sudden "Eureka!" type of discovery which quickly flashes before the consciousness and goes away, being replaced by the feeling of energy running through the body and nourishing the mind and spirit.

Lu Dongbin is using Laozi's concept of non-action being a *yin*, or female activity, and action is being a *yang*, or male activity. Because *yin* and *yang* constantly turn into and give way to each other, then the state of non-action becoming active is a requisite goal of Daoist meditation.

To become genuinely active and put the intention of the body and mind into the process would be less beneficial than to allow the body and mind to simply adjust naturally to the movement of energy occurring from stillness.

Huo Yuanji also said:

"Before the division of heaven and earth, the way was hung in the turbid centre of emptiness. After heaven and earth became sovereign, the way was not harmed."

This is an explanation of the quiet and non-judgemental way in which nature simply goes between action and non-action. Daoists view non-action and quiet as being the genuine route to achieving the correct circulation of energy and illumination of the mind.

So, "know the ancestral progenitor" is a way of saying that to understand the relationship between quiet and movement, *yin* and *yang*, and *wuwei* and *wei wu wei*, is to understand the root of all beings. Typically in Daoism, to discuss the ancestor actually means that we are talking about that which gives birth to all things: silent emptiness. In this case, the ancestral progenitor refers to the way the universe is before anything happens. This may be at the time of creation of the universe, or before the body is born into the world, or before a thought or feeling enters the mind.

This is again related to the *yin yun* state of primordial chaos, for it is from silence and chaos from which all being emerges.

Even in the Chinese understanding of Christianity, it is said, "First was the *Dao*, and the *Dao* gave birth to all things." We can see by this that in China, the *Dao* is the great progenitor of all things but does not exist of itself, but rather occurs beyond existence and nonexistence. It silently governs all things and is beyond all understanding. To return to quiet and know the ancestral progenitor is. in a sense, the closest we can get to the truth of nature. The mind must be held without judgment or desire, and it will eventually simply revert back to its own nature.

Without event for who knows how long?

This passage of the poem simply refers to the idea that the *wu wei* state should be held on to indefinitely during meditation practice. There is not a set correct time for the mind to be inactive, but rather, the amount of time staying within the deep meditative state is decided naturally by the body rather than by the intention of the person practicing. This idea is in keeping with the later Daoist belief that "the mystery gate," or the aperture through which the non-action state is entered, does not occur in any fixed physical location but rather appears spontaneously during meditation practice and is subject to random change without obvious cause.

Laozi refers to this as "Long the people will be without knowing or desire. He who knows this has no motive to be brave. Acting without action, he has no rules to be fettered by."

People who understand the non-action state will know that the mind is an essentially transient phenomenon and, whether one is with or without thought, this state will naturally yield and give away to another, which of itself will ultimately change continuously and without stop.

That which is eternally real must accord with nature.

Lu Dongbin viewed emptiness as the only true and eternal event. Anything which comes into existence will always eventually perish and, as such, is transient and unimportant. Emptiness as the great root of reality, from which all being emerges, therefore, is the true nature of all things.

Lu believed that the elixir of immortality could be obtained by according with the quiet and empty nature of reality and resting perpetually there. One of the key facets of Daoism is the study of how emptiness may be applied to life. Laozi says the best way to know the *Dao* is to day by day subtract from one's knowledge of the world. More precisely, the only way to understand the mind is to not assume that one already understands the nature of mind. In short, Lu Dongbin and Laozi are both suggesting that the non-action state must eventually merge with the natural world.

This activity may be accomplished simply by remaining in a state of quiet emptiness and not moving from it. The practice must be treated as an ongoing thing, and just like reading, writing, and riding a bike, it is something that improves with practice.

Eventually, when the non-action state becomes a natural response of the body to the action of sitting in meditation, then one will be able to gradually merge with nature. It is extremely common for meditators to have experiences such as melding with the room around them and losing sense of their physical self. Haung Yuanji referred to this as "no me, no self, and a genuine, real, original human existence."

The idea that a human being may exist without being conscious of self is a key to understanding the reasons for meditation. Just as in the preceding passage—"without activity for who knows how long"—we must be willing to not even know ourselves in order to truly benefit from the non-action state.

The secret of conforming to nature is to not become lost.

Although we wish to occupy a selfless state and rest without action, we must also keep in mind not to fall into a trance or fall asleep while meditating. The greatest benefit can be taken from meditation when the perceptive part of our consciousness is accompanying the practice. Laozi used the concept of *Dao de* or "observation of the way" to explain this. Keeping in mind that *Dao* refers to a way which is travelled but which is not knowable and *de* as being the process by which we observe thoughts and emotions, then we cannot completely disappear into the way if our goal is to really understand and benefit from it. *De* as a character is made up of a radical which indicates humanity, and an eye above a heart. This means the character indicates the way in which people observe and understand their emotions. The Chinese interpretation of heart is closely related to the emotional mind and the mind which has desire and takes action. Laozi believed that if people observe their minds closely, they can make great strides in achieving a higher level of consciousness. Lu Dongbin expanded on this idea by explaining that the concept of non-action must be accompanied by presence of mind. This is a silent presence and does not involve contemplation of anything aside from observation of the inner body, but it does imply that we do not lose consciousness during practice.

Not lost, the mind will settle itself.

When the mind is directed to stillness and kept there without disappearing, it will naturally cause the senses to relax and enter a deep, natural state which Daoists call *zhen Yi* or "the true mind." This state is one in which conscious thought is not emphasized and is open, free, and unfettered by the outside world.

The mind at rest, the qi returning to itself.

Daoists believe that when the mind slows down and stops, the body has time to regulate the flow of breath and energy on its own. In a more modern sense, we can consider the concept that during deep sleep, the Central Nervous system halts most activity and the Parasympathetic nervous system takes up the work of repairing the body. Just as the Parasympathetic Nervous System cannot be autonomously controlled, so Daoists believe that in order to control the energy of the body, people must first give up control of the mind.

This concept has two important factors, the first is that in order to breathe better, it is important to let the breath come and go in a smooth and unimpeded way, this type of breathing is the same as that which occurs when looking at a calm lake or a beautiful nature scene. This breathing does not require any active participation on the part of the brain and nervous system, it simply regulates itself. The second concept is that when the mind is relaxed to the point at which it settles, the sensation of an electrical energy in the body begins to naturally spread to all parts. This energy is what the Daoists call *qi* or the natural energy that pulses through the body when meditation practice enters a deep state. This stage can only happen after passing through "the mystery gate," which is the stage of practice in which the mind clicks over from being autonomously controlled to being mostly regulated by the automatic action of the peripheral nervous system.

Even though the mind is completely at rest, there is an alert and attentive feeling and the breath becomes natural and free. Lu Dongbin believed that if the mind were placed deep in the abdomen for a long time, and the breathing were to become stable, then it would be possible for the mind, the body, and the energy to return to their natural state, rather than the world of thoughts and ideas.

The qi returning will cause elixir to form itself.

After the breath circulates naturally for long enough, a different sensation may begin to occur.

This sensation is a strong, healing feeling that circulates from the abdomen through the entire body.

Some effects that are common during this phase of practice are to feel as though the spine and skull become free, the muscles deeply relax, and the body has sensation everywhere.

The concept of Elixir in Daoism is related to the idea that "returning to the root and going back to the origin is the king of medicine." The idea at play is still representative of the nervous system relaxing and regulating itself. The thoughts during this time hold no practical reason, and the mind, although it may not be without thought, it clear and unbothered. The breathing becomes extremely comfortable and often the person practising may experience sensations of the entire body being filled with light, or even the feeling of disappearing into the room. It is also possible during this time to experience vision states, but these states should be treated merely as a side effect of practice, rather than holding any specific spiritual meaning.

In the centre of the boiler is the marriage of water and fire.

Lu Dongbin believed that the centre of the body, behind the navel, is the genuine root of life.

He said in the poem *Six Phrase Decree, "until the day you die, stir fire and water in the brewing pot."*

In this case, the brewing pot refers to the lower *Dantian*, the energetic centre in the abdomen where Daoists believe the majority of the pre-natal or "raw" energy of the body resides.

The concept of stirring fire and water refers to the mind (represented as fire, a lively element that causes action to occur) being directed toward the centre of the lower abdomen, which is considered to be where the water element resides in the body. The fire and water, when mixed, are considered to create a natural steam in the body that can circulate freely, relaxing the muscles and mind and putting the body in a deep state of rest.

The Daoists also believe that water and fire represents that harmony of *Yin* and *Yang*. Lv Dongbin used many different paired phrases such as water and fire, dragon and tiger, and so on. These phrases refer to several different ways in which *yin* and *yang* can be practiced in the body to create "*taiji*," or "the harmony of *yin* and *yang*."

When water and fire are correctly paired through conscious engagement with the empty space in the lower abdomen, it is possible to become ever calmer and eventually to enter the state of "non-action," which Lu Dongbin refers to at the start of the poem.

Yin and Yang born, they return and revert.

Lu believed that the stage after this was to naturally allow *yin* and *yang* to give birth to and arise in each other. In Daoist philosophy, *yin* and *yang* harmonize together in such a way that they are always changing between each other and merging together in different ways. The action should be smooth and continuous in nature, and so it is considered important to remain natural during meditation in order to allow the energy of the body to naturally change between *yin* and *yang*, rather than to purposefully adjust the level of the intensity of the energetic feeling. An easier way to understand this is just to allow the energetic feeling of the body to move wherever it wants to, naturally, and without emotional interference.

Another way of understanding *yin* and *yang* in meditation is that when the breath goes out, it is labelled as *yang*, because it is active, moving upward and outward. The in breath is considered as *yin*, because it moves inward and downward, toward the earth, which represents pure *yin* energy.

Huang Yuanji said that to master the movement of *yin* and *yang* in the breath could help the mind revert to the state of "no extermity," or a condition of total stillness and relaxation.

Everything transforms into one clap of thunder.

This concept is that once *yin* and *yang* have been harmonized for long enough, the body will suddenly enter the *xian tian* or "pre-heaven" state in which the body suddenly feels a sensation of total circulation of energy in every part. This can also be accompanied by sound, or sudden feelings of surging sensations all through the torso, legs, and head, as well as the arms, hands, and feet.

This state is the true aim of Daoist cultivation as it is the time when the body begins to truly regulate itself and is no longer dependent on outside stimulus delivered to the Central Nervous System. The body is able to relax, and Huang Yuanji called this state, "one hundred meridians flow connected."

White clouds gather over the morning peak.

"White clouds gathering over the morning peak" refers to the feeling of being surrounded by *qi* and having a thin layer of energy everywhere in the body, just like clouds hanging over a mountain.

It can also be seen to mean the state of *ming shen* or "far away and distant." This feeling is the period at which the mind begins to divert away from consciously-driven thought and goes into an unclear, remote, and non-logical state. *Ming shen* directly predates going into the pre-birth phase of meditation, which is the central goal in Daoist meditation. Sometimes the area around the top of the head can feel as though there is a great deal of energy inside and all around.

The sweet syrup wine must be bursting.

The sweet syrup here refers to a very early Chinese variety of tea called *gan lu* or "dew drop." This reference in the case of meditation is quite similar to the Buddhist idea of clarified butter being similar to a clear and stable mind. A physical effect of meditation is to make it feel as though there is a fullness and sense of clarity in the mind. This can also manifest as a feeling of concentration of a strong, positive feeling in the head and behind the eyes. This type of feeling can also occur in the entire body and can open and spill over into a complete sense of awareness of *qi* energy. When the *qi* energy is so full it seems bursting, then this is considered to be "sweet syrup."

Drink all of your long-life alcohol.

At this phase in the practice, it may seem like a genuine feeling of health and longevity has emerged in the body. Lu Dongbin refers to this as "long-life alcohol," and this passage in the poem refers to the concept that you should rest in this feeling as long as possible. People of Lu's time may not have had a very well developed method of describing the effects of meditation, and so it is not surprising that he referred to the effects as being similar to being drunk. This feeling is a kind of like drunkenness without becoming stupid. It almost seems as though the self no longer exists, and yet one is not asleep. The real mind remains, but nothing else exists.

So free and unfettered, who could know?

Meditation is a gradual method by which one may enter into a more open, free, relaxed existence. As the mind becomes silent, it also becomes more relaxed, and it feels as though the ties which bond us to the world all disappear. My teacher, Yang Hai, referred to the feeling after meditation by saying "It is so nice! I could never feel angry or have any negative judgement about the world after meditating." This sense of freedom can be achieved directly and is not a philosophy or ephemeral concept. Simply focus on non-action until the mind becomes calm, generates the feeling of energy and then of longevity. From there, simply stay with the feeling and gradually become free and unfettered.

Sometimes when we meditate, it is possible to feel as though there is music playing, although one is in complete silence. The philosopher Zhuangzi said, "You hear the music of the flutes, but can you hear the music of the earth? You can hear the music of the earth, but can you hear the music of the heavens?" This exceptional awareness of the nature of the world is a by-product of meditation. If we hold no judgement, then everything we hear or see will seem new to us.

The simple sound of silence in the room, when we truly recognize it, may seem like music to the ears.

Sit and listen to the music without strings.
Brightness meets with the beginning of good fortune.

Once meditation practice has entered the pre-birth phase, or the phase after non-action changes into action without action, then it is quite common for the nature of the mind to become illuminated. This light may be of various colours or may be accompanied by mental images, but typically this feeling is associated with deep calm, happiness, and a feeling of profound positivity.

Even though at this part of practice, you may feel like you want to go and do something active and positive, you should just remain seated with the feeling and gradually transform it back into silence and calm. This has a very beneficial effect on the mind and can cause the body to gradually let go of tension carried in the muscles and nervous system.

Practice this a total of twenty times.

This phrase simply means that you should practice for a long time. Even though the basic idea is that the *yuan jing* energetic state should flow around the body in a circular fashion multiple times, it is important to recognize that after a certain period of practice, the circulation feeling will no longer occur, and it will simply become a united feeling of complete energy and vitality in the body. "Practice this a total of twenty times," therefore, simply means to stay in the meditation state for as long as possible.

Another traditional way to say this is, "Practice for the length of three incense sticks," which usually means about an hour and a half. Actually, there is no correct amount of practice, and you should just practice as much as you can while still gaining benefit. If you practice too much, you may lose some of the benefit at first, since you will exclude other elements from your daily life. Even practicing for five minutes is better than not practicing.

This is the method of climbing a ladder to heaven.

Lu Dongbin believed that meditation was a way to become liberated from the "red dust" of the world. Red dust refers to the concept of the thoughts which distract us from the actual experience of being alive. Lu believed that the basic nature of the world is good but people get lost in their thoughts and desires, and so are not able to enjoy life as much as they could. In this way, meditation, which clears the mind and improves the energy, can be seen as the ladder to heaven, even though one is still alive on the earth.

CHAPTER 11:

POST BIRTH DAOIST HEALTH PRESERVATION TECHNIQUES

Although the main premise of this book is to introduce Daoist meditation techniques which essentially work according to the pre-heaven or static approach to cultivating life energy, it is also important to briefly discuss other ways in which Daoists cultivate themselves outside of seated meditation practice.

Many people have heard the term *qigong* before but maybe are not completely clear about the history of this term and what exactly it means.

To help simplify out discussion, we should look at *qigong* as being a modern style of synthesized exercise based on ancient Daoist, Buddhist, and Medical methods of Chinese health protection practices. *Qigong*, as such, is essentially any exercise or set of exercises which is used to improve the *qi* energy of the human body. These exercises typically involve movement, stretching, and visualization

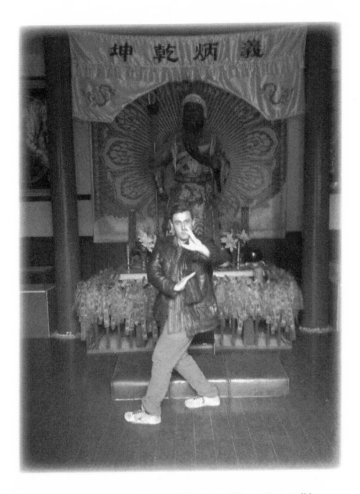

Baguazhang in front of a statue of Guanyu: The author striking "dragon stretches its claws," a posture from the popular Chinese internal martial art of baguazhang. The statue behind him is of Guanyu, the famous Chinese general who has been deified by both Daoists and Buddhists alike.

of energy in order to produce the desired effect of causing the blood and *qi* to flow effortlessly around within the body, healing it.

Qigong as we know it now was essentially an invention of the Chinese Communist Party, which, during the 1950s and 1960s, was not able to provide comprehensive medical care to all people in the Republic. As such, many different types of exercise such as taijiquan, Daoist yoga, self-massage, and even some types of meditation techniques were compiled into a series of exercises designed to prevent degeneration of the body and in some cases, stand in when medicine was not available.

Although the term *qigong* is a relatively new one, exercises developed to strengthen the energy of the body have existed in China for thousands of years. These exercises have many names such as *daoyin* (Daoist yoga), *neigong* (internal exercise), *baduanjin* (Eight Brocade exercise), and so on. Some are more effective at developing energy while others are better for stretching the connective tissue and strengthening the body.

In any event, all of these exercises work on a principle called the *hou tian*, or "post-birth principle." In this sense, this is where the key difference between Dan Dao Meditation and *qi gong* occurs. While *dan dao* is an essentially silent and non-moving practice, *qigong* and more ancient varieties of health exercise are what would be commonly considered as requiring physical and mental effort.

Qigong style exercises also tend to view *qi* energy as being more in line with Chinese medicine theory, in that the *qi* is considered to move with the blood through the veins, arteries, capillaries, and along with the breath and heartbeat. This idea of *qi* is dramatically different from the Daoist interpretation, which holds that *qi* occurs as a manifestation of concentration on emptiness (or in a more modern sense, that *qi* occurs because of the relationship between the mind, the autonomous nervous system, and the endocrine system). Because of this, *qigong* and *dan dao* have dramatically different results.

Typically, *dan dao* is used to pursue higher realms of consciousness and to heal the body and mind of flaws associated with both impure thoughts and the wear and tear associated with day to day life.

Qigong is more associated with assisting in the regulation of blood flow throughout the body, flushing the lymphatic system, and giving one the feeling of free and healthy breathing and heartbeat. This is a dramatic over simplification of the benefits of both *qi gong* and *dan dao*, but by now, you should be able to understand that there is a difference between these two very complimentary exercises.

In this section, I will introduce three ancient post-birth health cultivation exercises from the Daoist health classic, *Yang Sheng Lei Yao*, or "The Method of Cultivating Better Health." These translations will be accompanied by explanations when required and photographs when appropriate.

YANG SHENG HEALTH CULTIVATION EXERCISES

1: Water Tide Clears Away Future Troubles

- ❖ *Each morning when you awake,*
- ❖ *sit upright and focus on the feeling of breathing.*
- ❖ *Touch the tongue to the roof of the mouth,*
- ❖ *close the mouth, and breathe freely.*
- ❖ *Let the saliva naturally form until the mouth is full.*
- ❖ *Swallow it in three sections and focus on delivering it downward.*
- ❖ *After much practice, the five organs will not be scorched by evil fire,*
- ❖ *the four limbs will all fill naturally with blood and energy,*
- ❖ *diseases will not occur, allowing you to clear away future troubles*
- ❖ *and grow old without becoming weak.*

This piece has several concepts from Chinese medicine as important aspects of its practice.

Basically, the idea is that when you wake up in the morning, it is very easy for the mind to become overwhelmed. The nervous system has not had time to acclimatize to doing activities other than sleeping, and it is easy to become angry, or develop what is described here as "evil fire." The meaning of evil fire is related to the mind being easy to enrage and to the nervous system being damaged by being shocked into action without any time to naturally reset.

The goal of this exercise is to use the cooling benefits of developing saliva in the mouth and swallowing it, while being focused on breathing evenly and calmly. These two things, combined with the natural relaxation of sitting up in bed, can allow the practitioner to ease into the waking state and set a trend of relaxation and calm for the whole first part of his or her day. This practice combines the idea of soft meditation techniques, such as feeling the breath, with the Chinese medicine idea that the saliva contains many beneficial cooling aspects when partitioned as swallowed gradually and with purpose.

2: Lift the fire to grasp eternal peace

❖ *Around the second hour of noon,*

❖ *Place your mind on the real fire of the yongchuan point of the feet.*

- *First, move the left foot toward the jade pillow, past the mud ball, and to the dan tian a total of three times.*

- *Repeat this on the right side, and then do the exercise again, past the wei lu a total of three times.*

- *After a long time, this will warm the hundred meridians and cause the energy to smoothly flow to the organs.*

- *With no sluggishness in the four limbs, the bones of the body will be strengthened.*

The term *zi wu* means "something which occurs in the middle of the day between 11am and 1pm." This is considered to be the time of day when the body is at the peak of genuine *yang* energy and, as such, is a very important time to practice self-cultivation. This very easy exercise uses the point at the bottom of the foot as a place to set the intention. This point, called *yongchuan*, is considered to be the way in which the *qi* of the body connects to the earth. It is associated with the leg meridian called the *yinqiao*, which flows smoothly from the lower *dantian*, in the abdominal area.

This exercise is meant to be used as a way to connect these three important points and develop a smooth flow of blood and oxygen through the lower body.

The "jade pillow," refers to the point where the spine connects with the skull on the back of the head. To move the leg toward the jade pillow simply means that the leg should be moved upward.

During the first three repetitions on each side, you should emphasize moving the knee up to the *dantian*, and gradually lowering the foot back to the floor. This is followed by repeating the same exercise, but this time, focusing on the "*wei lu*" point, which is associated with the deep abdominal muscles near the rectum and internal part of the anus. The idea of the second set of repetitions is to exercise the deeper aspect of the abdomen and the organs associated with excretion and reproduction.

The first aspect of the exercise is believed to massage the organs in the digestive system and to mildly augment the breathing and heartbeat.

This exercise is also good for balance, proprioceptive ability (the ability to feel things in the area outside of your body), and, possibly, for flushing the lymphatic system, which is located near the inguinal fold in the inner leg.

3: Protect the dreams from being lost and seal the golden cabinet

The desire to move can infuriate scorching fire, scorching fire can make the spirit tired, a tired spirit will make the essence and bones weak, and you will lose energy during dreaming. At the time between being fully awake and sleeping, breathe evenly and focus the mind and spirit, glide the left hand over the umbilical area 14 times, and repeat with the right hand. Move the two hands up and down the torso from the waist to just above the arm pits and focus on the energy there for a total of 14 repetitions, finally placing the hands on the dantian, breathing lightly until comfortable, and then turning on your side, with knees together in fetal position until you fall asleep.

The Daoists believe that when we dream in our sleep, we can lose much *qi* energy and that it is important to seal the energy in the body before going to sleep. This practice is to build up a wall of post-birth energy and then seal it in by laying in the fetal position while focusing on the *dantian* and legs. This practice pulls awareness away from the head, and, as such, makes it easier to get to sleep without staying awake thinking. It is a great remedy to insomnia caused by thinking too much, or excessive caffeine intake from drinking coffee.

PRACTICAL DAN DAO: USING MEDITATION IN LIFE

One major issue for people who want to meditate seriously is that they often lead busy lives and aren't sure how to make enough time to practice. This can seem overwhelming and can cause stress and confusion about how to prioritize one's time. In this section, I want to help describe some ways in which you can optimize practice time without eating into your otherwise busy schedule. Making time where there doesn't seem to be any is a great way to make quick progress, as well as help you to live a more relaxed, energetic, and happy life.

1: Meditate at the office.

Many people who work at desk jobs don't realize just how much time is spent between tasks.

There are always a few minutes in a day when one is playing video games, looking at websites, waiting for something to print and so on. This is a great time to sit down, focus calmly on your centre, and quiet your mind. Even just a few minutes of meditation can help you to "recharge" and approach the rest of the day with poise and calm.

It is even possible to use meditation principles while you walk from place to place, go to get a coffee, or use the washroom. Simply focus the attention on pushing the "energy," feeling downward into your abdomen and through your legs into the ground. This very mild activity can be done virtually any time, and it qualifies as a type of very powerful qi gong practice, which can help strengthen your energy and make you feel more connected with your body and mind while you work.

2: Meditate after exercise.

Have you ever noticed that after you exercise or do sports, you tend to be able to feel the blood flowing through your body more evenly? Is your breathing smoother and deeper?

Daoists consider this to be "post-heaven energy," the type of energy which is cultivated by doing healthy physical activities. This energy is considered to be the oxygen which moves in the blood, and is effective in making you healthier and more connected to your body.

This can be further improved by focusing on doing a short meditation directly after exercise.

This meditation can be done seated or standing, and you can simply focus the mind on your lower *dantian* (The space about an inch below and inch inside of your navel) and allow the post-heaven energy feeling to gradually collect there. After it has collected for a long time, it will gradually begin to refine itself into a deeper, more restful, pre-heaven energy, which can naturally circulate through the whole body. This is one way to use physical activity to cultivate real, long lasting benefits on the energetic systems of the body.

Typically, if this exercise is done standing, it will be most useful to collect the circulating energy in the *dantian*. If the practice is done seated, with the eyes closed, there is a chance to go into the state of "non-action," and enter the mystery gate. It is your choice about how deep you want to go, but it is a great idea to use the good energy you have collected and cultivate it into a powerful, subliminal energy in the body.

USING DAOIST PRINCIPLES IN OTHER AREAS OF LIFE

The kind of practice described above can work for virtually any kind of activity, but it is also important to recognize that Daoist practice can extend to anything and is not restricted only to silent meditation. Even though the ultimate goal of Daoist practice is to observe non-action and cultivate stillness, it is still very common for Daoists to do physical exercise, art, writing, music, and many other types of culture while using the skills they have learned through meditation on silence.

One of the greatest gifts of Daoism to the world is the idea that each individual part of life makes up the totality of life. If you use this principle to live by, it can make it so that there are no parts of your life which are out of cooperation with other parts of your life. Using this method, you can apply the skills of meditation to virtually anything!

HOW DAOIST PHILOSOPHY WORKS IN DAY TO DAY LIFE

Daoist meditation practice is not independent of a mindset and does not occur by itself.

All of Daoism, be it the philosophy, religion, or practice, cropped up around the original texts of Laozi and Zhuangzi, who taught a type of non-judgemental non-differentiation of reality.

Basically, both authors advocated the idea that if one is to truly appreciate reality as an experience, rather than as a thoughtful observation of experience, it would be required that one were able to view the experience as it occurred rather than holding pre-conceived ideals about how the experience ought to unfold.

This philosophy of non-judgement is principle in the mastery of meditation, as meditation is an essentially silent and non-active practice. The skill of not differentiating things in our thoughts as being either good or bad can be carried over into every part of life and be of great psychological help. If we can learn to tap into the root of what we believe to be good or bad, right or wrong, comfortable or uncomfortable, and deeply understand it, then there is room for immense personal growth. Imagine if it were possible to transcend the belief that you are not able to do certain things. Imagine being willing to learn new skills without the fear of failure. A state of relaxed and quiet non-judgement can help us obtain these skills and make them our own.

Try it now, don't wait! Stand, sit, or lie down, and don't focus on anything in particular. Hold this feeling for a while and then get up and observe the room around you. Is anything different? Are you able to let go of some of your assumptions about the world around you?

Now try engaging in a physical activity that you are not completely comfortable doing.

This could be something like playing a sport with which you are not intimately acquainted, or else something as simple as standing for an extended period of time on one leg. Whatever the task, be it physical or emotional, simply putting yourself into the state of non-judgement and emotional calm can greatly assist you in your day to day life.

A FINAL THOUGHT.

The practice of elixir Daoism is a very long and assiduous process. There are at least 500 books in the Daoist canon on the subject of meditation, and very few people alive today have read all of them.

As such, there is not enough room to fit every concept in elixir practice into one book. With luck, people may find this work useful and gain some insight into creating a healthy and bountiful practice for themselves. Those who are already experienced may be able to shed new light on their practice and go deeper than before.

This book was written with the express intention of sharing the genuine practice of Daoist meditation with people as openly and freely as possible. It is my desire to help others to find the deep level of calm and longevity that Daoists have known for so many generations.

I hope in reading this book you have been able to decipher the basics of meditation practice. Make sure you go back to review each section to check your progress.

The goal of meditation does not have to be complete enlightenment, removing oneself from the wheel of karma, or attributing practice to any religious or superstitious belief. Just as the great 20th century master Chen Yingning said, *"Daoism is simply the study of the use of emptiness."* The correct practice of meditation on emptiness can yield a result which makes us feel more full and gives our lives more meaning. This great medicine for both mind and body should be pursued with diligence and a pure heart. What I have introduced in this book is the foundational theory of Daoist meditation and is sufficient to master the basics. I hope in the future to release more books, each one going more deeply into the specific practices of different Daoist schools throughout Chinese history.

When practicing Daoism, we must not consider our attainment as finished, but instead attempt to gain new insight into the nature of our being each and every day. If you are feeling tired, or ill, I hope that the practices in this book will help to make you feel better. If you already feel good, I hope you will use this opportunity to conserve it and save your positive energy in order to grow old in a graceful and happy way.

Although meditation is not the answer to all of life's problems, it can help us shine a light on how to solve them – and with great effort and honesty, can help people develop into more complete persons.

The mountain is very tall and the path is often not clear,
and even if you do not make it all the way to the top,
you should persevere and not give up.
In this way, you may find newness and life in each
waking breath.

Thank you for reading this book, and if you find the practices in it useful, please practice them seriously as often as possible.

APPENDIX:

DAOIST HISTORY

Toward the end of the Zhou dynasty periods of Chinese Spring and Autumn, there was an explosion of philosophy in Chinese thought. Of the hundred schools of philosophy, two stood out above all others. The teachings of Confucius became the core of Chinese social behaviour, being composed of practical ideals and reverence for seniority. Daoism represented the dynamic aspect of Chinese thought, or, more accurately, the aspect of Chinese philosophy which could not be used as a formula by which to conduct ceremonies, or make laws.

The first Daoist philosopher, Laozi, was famous for leaving behind the treatise known as *Dao De Jing* or "The Way of Virtue Classic." This book used very open language to illustrate the concept that it is not possible to accurately predict the nature of reality.

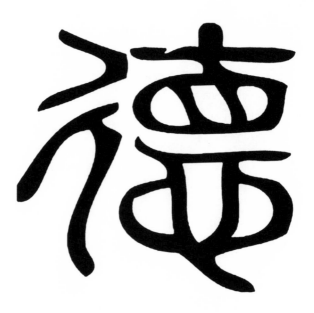

De, the Daoist concept of Virtue: The Chinese pictograph, De, is considered by most to signify virtuous behavior, or the virtuous quality of a person or persons. In fact, this much earlier reading of the character shows its original meaning, which is related to observation. The left most radical is made up of the picture of a person, while the top right is a human eye, and the bottom right is the character for heart. Together, this infers that people with virtue must be ever observant of their emotions and not act rashly. The eye over the heart symbolizes one's ability to control oneself simply by knowing oneself. Laozi said, "To be victorious over others is to be called powerful. To be victorious over oneself is to be called strong."

LAOZI

Laozi most likely lived between the 6th and 4th Century B.C. and was the librarian of the Zhou Dynasty court. There are many stories about him and his wisdom, but all that is known for sure is that the classic "*Dao De Jing*" is attributed to him

Although all stories about Laozi are at best contained within the realm of legend, it is often considered to be accurate that upon retiring from the Zhou court, Laozi was urged to leave behind a recording of his philosophy to benefit future generations.

Laozi's main teaching can be summed up as "The map is not the territory," "It is better to remain silent than to speak and endanger oneself," and "to live according to kindness and positivity."

Many people assume that Laozi was writing to a prince of the Zhou court, but some historians have inferred Laozi's message to apply directly to common people, while using political terminology to explain his spiritual precepts.

In the Daoist religion, Laozi is considered as the head of the Gods.

Although there are many stories about Laozi, it is also possible that his book was in fact written by many different people. This is backed up by the fact that there are multiple different historical versions of the *Dao De Jing*

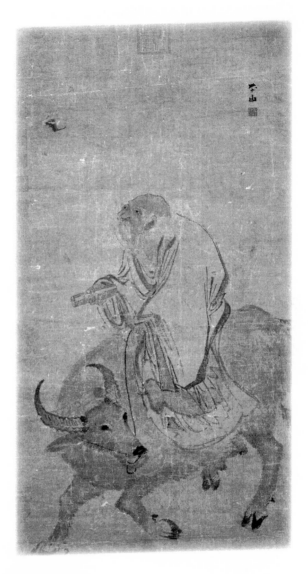

Tang dynasty depiction of the philosopher Laozi riding West on an Ox.

which have been found on ancient scrolls dating back as far as the Han Dynasty, around 1 AD.

Each of the versions, although similar in meaning, contains many different arrangements of characters, chapters, and ideas.

The easiest way to understand the *Dao De Jing* and Laozi is simply to read as many different versions as possible and think about it deeply.

After the time of Laozi, several other philosophers appeared of whom the most important was Zhuangzi. It is important to know here that Laozi and Zhuangzi most likely did not know each other, but they carried similar opinions about the nature of the world and human interaction.

Zhuangzi wrote a series of stories that criticized the regimented nature of the Chinese government system and suggested that following the rules of society would only make people perverted and unhappy. Zhuangzi put great effort into creating a contextual document for people to understand that their understanding of the world and the actual nature of the world are not the same. Unlike Laozi, Zhuangzi was a story-teller and preferred to illustrate his points by making examples of other people and their relationship with nature.

Zhuangzi was also more clearly an advocate of meditation than Laozi and told several stories about people meditating in nature and coming to an understanding of how the world works by simply observing the world around them. Although the work of Laozi can be applied directly to meditation practice, Zhuangzi was the first writer in Daoism to specifically make reference to seated meditation practices.

ZHUANGZI'S MEDITATION

This selection from Zhuangzi shows how he conceptualized meditation as simply being a method of observing nature and explains the concept of using the body as if were a large ear capable of hearing the sounds of wind as they gust past one's quietly seated form.

Nanguo Ziqi leaned back as he sat, looked at the sky, and sighed. He seemed lost to the world and not noticing his companion. Yancheng Ziyou stood a while, facing him, and asked, "Why do you sit so? Your form looks like withered wood, and your aspect like dead ashes. You sit today leaned back like this, and yet it is also not you sitting here.

Ziqi said: "Desist! You don't know what is good, and yet you ask! Today I lost myself, how can you know?

You have heard the sound of manmade pipes, but do you hear the pipes of the earth? You hear the pipes of the earth, but you don't hear the pipes of heaven."

Ziyou said, "May I ask where they come from?"

Ziqi replied, "The great piercing sound of the screaming, is that not called the wind? This is only coming from emptiness, and, like this, it blows through the ten thousand oracles as an angry hiss.

Yet this is not the only sound of the wind, is it?

Although Laozi and Zhuangzi were not the only Daoist writers of the time, they were the most important. Some other writers included Liezi and Yuzi, who both wrote books according to their interpretation of Laozi's core concepts. Neither of these writers is as important to the history of Daoism as the works of Laozi and Zhuangzi's, which set down the essential theory of Daoism and were used in all later Daoist works to provide a back bone for practice.

After the end of the Spring and Autumn period, around 200 AD, Daoism experienced a shift in ideology as a group of rebels in Sichuan managed to overthrow the local government there and establish a kingdom which was ruled by a Daoist king. The king of this empire was named Zhang Daoling, and he is often credited as the founder of religious Daoism.

Zhang's Five Pecks of Rice movement offered people salvation from the frequent wars occurring at the time and a place in his kingdom of "Celestial Masters" in Sichuan, in return for a donation of rice to the cause.

ZHANG DAOLING AND THE DAOIST KINGDOM OF SICHUAN

Zhang Daoling, born Zhang Ling, was a minor political official from Jiangsu province. After he retired, he became a hermit and went into the wild to learn the way of self-cultivation. He is said to have seen a vision of Laozi, who told him that he should take a group of followers to Sichuan to create a kingdom based on righteous values and correct action.

He and his followers rebelled and overthrew the government in Sichuan, creating their own empire based on what Zhang believed to be Daoist virtues.

The kingdom focused on the value of self-cultivation through various types of exercise, chanting, playing music, performing rites, and so on, but frowned on offering animal sacrifices and generally abstained from sexual activity except for reproductive purposes.

Although it is generally agreed that Zhang Daoling was the first leader of a Daoist religion, it is also considered probable that he simply appropriated early folk religious practices and added Daoist deities and ideals as the base for his religion.

The empire in Sichuan only lasted three generations, at which point it was ceded back to China under the rule of military commander Cao Cao. Because Zhang's descendants cooperated with Cao Cao, their religion was made the national religion of China during that time.

There are no documents surviving from the era of Zhang's kingdom in Sichuan, but the popular Daoist commentary "*Xiang Er*" is often ascribed to Zhang Daoling, although it is hotly contested among scholarship circles.

After the time of Zhang Daoling, Daoism underwent several changes, principally in that it fell into disuse to some extent until the Wei dynasty, in about 400 CE. During the Wei there came about a group of literary scholars who engaged in a type of literary criticism of philosophical documents named "real talk."

The real talk group wrote many treatises explaining the inner meaning of Laozi and the divination book the "*Yi Jing.*" Among the most famous of these thinkers was Wang Bi who argued that Laozi's "*Daode Jing*" is a book based on the study of emptiness. Wang Bi asserted that Laozi's concept of non-action as a way of doing things naturally was the central theory that held the book together. Wang's treatise became recognized as one of the most important theoretical commentaries of the "*Daode Jing.*"

WANG BI, BOY GENIUS

Wang Bi was a scholar of Daoism who helped to create "The Mystery Study School of Daoism," which is often referred to by western scholars as Neo-Daoism. He famously wrote a commentary on the "*Daode Jing*" as well as the "*Yijing*," an important early book on Chinese divination.

Wang Bi wrote the bulk of his work when he was very young and died of illness at twenty-three years of age. Wang asserted that the "*Daode Jing*" and "*Yijing*" were connected in theory and that the inner meaning of Daoist philosophy was related to the cosmological concept that emptiness is the root of all reality.

Wang Bi, despite his young age, is considered as one of the most important philosophical writers in Chinese history. His ideas strongly influenced Daoism in its later permutations as a philosophy, religion, and practice.

Wang Bi's work was accompanied by Guo Xiang who wrote an important commentary on Zhuangzi, which later became one of the most standard ways by which to view his work.

Together, their Mystery Study School promoted the ideals of Daoism as philosophy and allowed the continuation of Daoist thought outside the framework of a religious practice.

Although the development of the Celestial Masters movement and the Mystery Study School were at similar periods of Chinese history, it appears as if they were not connected deeply.

To some extent, this validates the ongoing assertion that Daoism is split into philosophical and religious practice. A further development, albeit later in history, was the foundation of the Zhong Lv Golden Elixir school of meditation. Essentially, a man named Lu Dongbin and his teacher, Han Zhongli, began to popularize the idea that Daoist meditation should be treated separately from other Daoist traditions. They felt that it was incorrect to practice external cultivation, which may have included things like chanting, praying, prostrations of various parts, and attempting to alter the body alchemically via the ingestion of metals such as mercury.

Previous to this, Daoism had experienced problems when some Daoist followers attempted to create an elixir of immortality by mixing various metals together and ingesting them as a potion.

Lu Dongbin had learned meditation from Han Zhongli and wrote a series of poems explaining how to practice meditation and why it was of benefit.

It should be noted that Lu and Han were not part of either the previous Daoist religion or philosophy movement and should be viewed as having created a unique

Daoist school of cultivation which is totally distinct from other methods.

LU FAMILY HUNDRED-WORD ANCESTOR TABLET

The most important writing to come out of the Zhong Lu meditation school was Lu Dongbin's hundred-character poem called "Lu Family Hundred-Word Ancestor Tablet."

The poem is a guide to meditation which uses the philosophy of Laozi to explain the method by which health can be achieved and the mind can be made calm.

It reads:

To cultivate energy, forget to say observe
direct the heart to acting without action
become quiet to know the ancestors
without activity who knows how long
to become immortal, you must correspond with nature
corresponding of nature you must not become lost
not being lost the mind will rest in itself
the mind resting, the energy will return to itself
the qi returning will naturally create medicine
inside the pot is the marriage of water and fire
yin and yang mutually return to each other
the world will change to the sound of one clap of thunder
white clouds gather over the morning peak

the sweet dew liquor must be full
drink your longevity alcohol
so free, who else could know?
Sit and listen to the music without strings
brightness and happiness will become your nature
repeat a total of twenty times
this is the way to find the ladder to heaven

The stories of Lu Dongbin and Han Zhongli point out the romance that is sometimes attached by Chinese people to the Daoist concept. It is said that Lu was a low level political official who was being frequently promoted and had a bright future. One night while he was cooking a pot of millet, he fell asleep. When he awoke from his dream, he went on with life as usual, climbing and climbing through the government until he reached a very high level of prestige. One day he encountered bad luck and lost everything. His wife betrayed him, and he was robbed by bandits, who ultimately stabbed him. As he lay dying, he awoke *from this dream* to be informed by his teacher, Han Zhongli, that he had played all of the characters of the dream in order to help Lu realize that fame and fortune were not the ultimate goal of life. In the story, Lu is said to have gone to study with Han for many years and eventually mastered the secrets of meditation.

However apocryphal these stories may seem, the grain of truth contained in them is that the practice of medi-

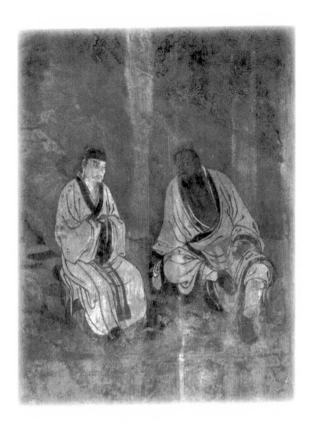

Lu Dongbin receiving instruction from Han Zhongli: Daoist immortals Lu Dongbin (left) and his teacher Han Zhongli (right) discuss the techniques of cultivating immortality in this Tang Song era painting.

tation may bring presence of mind that achievement and money cannot.

In religious Daoism, Lu Dongbin is considered as a very important God figure who can assist people in times of trouble. In meditation practice, Lu is considered as the progenitor of the internal elixir school, and Lu's teachings survive today in his own writings and also in those of the other masters of *Quanzhen* Daoism, such as Zhang Baoduan.

After Lu Dongbin's time, Daoism went into another relatively quiet period until around the time of Zhang Boduan. Zhang wrote the very important book "*Wuzhen Pian*" or "Understanding Reality." This book is the cornerstone of Daoist meditation classics and can be considered as the key classic of the Southern school of Daoism. "*Wuzhen Pian*" focuses on the cultivation of *Jindan*, or "golden elixir" through the practice of quiet meditation.

Zhang Boduan also helped to correct many misconceptions in Daoist practice, such as the ideas of using external methods of cultivation, including ingestion of potions and abandonment of all earthly ties in order to better cultivate the way. Zhang suggested that people simply follow the natural method of focusing deeply on calm and silence while allowing the body to attend to itself in a peaceful and non-judgemental way.

An important concept from "*Wuzhen Pian*" that lived into later Daoist ideas is "Use your full resolve to find the place from which the body originates. Return to the root and revert to the origin. This is the king of all medicine." This idea is that when the mind is placed deeply in the body, it is possible to return to and observe the root from which all life emerges. In another sense, this means people should focus themselves completely on the task of cultivating profound quiet and using the mind in this way can have a great and beneficial effect on the body and spirit.

"*Wuzhen Pian*" set the course for future events in Daoism and was pivotal to the foundation of the *Quanzhen* school. *Quanzhen* Daoism was founded by Wang Chongyang, a person who had planned a rebellion against Genghis Khan and claimed to have met Lu Dongbin and Han Zhongli, who taught him Daoist methods of self-cultivation. Wang, along with five students, went on to establish and formalize *Quanzhen* Daoist religious practice. *Quanzhen* Daoism is the current root of Daoist religion but also contains many practices such as *Taijiquan* and qigong which are used to help in the attainment of the *Dao*.

After the time of Zhang Baoduan came the foundation of the *Quanzhen* school of Daoism as taught by Wang Chongyang and his students. Wang was planning a rebellion against Genghis Khan when he supposedly met the immortals Lu Dongbin and Han Zhongli, who instructed him in the *Dao*. He went on to live for several years in a self-made tomb in the side of a mountain and met

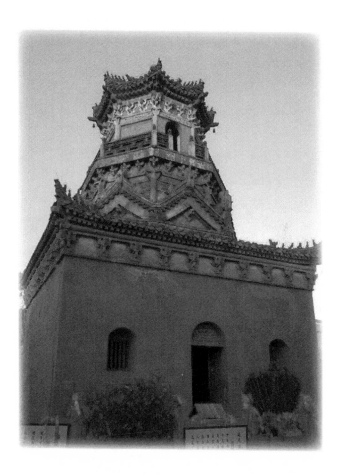

Quanzhen Daoist Temple Kaifeng City Henan: This temple dates back to the Yuan dynasty, around 1200 AD. At this time, Quanzhen Daoism was still in its early phases of development, but stood out as a type of Daoism which focused on the practical elements of Laozi's teachings. Quanzhen Daoists, such as Zhang Boduan and Huang Yuanji, believed that practice was the key to attaining a high level of skill in obtaining the Dao.

many students whom he taught about Daoism. Among his notable students was Chu Qiuji, who famously went to West China in order to beseech Genghis Khan to stop killing.

This was the time when Daoism was genuinely formalized as a religious practice, and the *Quanzhen* school of Daoist religion has the most clearly established group of gods and religious practices in the entire Daoist system.

During the time of the foundation of the *Quanzhen* school, Genghis Khan adopted Daoism as the state religion of China during the *Jin* Dynasty. After the fall of Khan, Daoism went on to flourish and temples were introduced to many Chinese towns and villages. The White Cloud Temple had already been established in Beijing, and Daoism became more popular all over China.

This carried on during the *Yuan*, *Ming*, and into the *Qing* dynasty, and the next important member in the Daoist group was the founder of the Middle School, Huang Yuanji.

HUANG YUANJI AND THE MIDDLE SCHOOL

No one is completely sure exactly when, but at some point during the late *Ming* or early *Qing* Dynasty, a man named Huang Yuanji penned an extremely important book called "*Daode Jing Chanwei*" or "Teaching Material of the *Daode Jing.*" This book is the only complete book to treat Laozi's philosophy as a method by which to meditate and achieve the Golden Elixir practice of cultivating health and longevity. Huang's book reads as an explanation of how Laozi's theory applies to meditation and how to correctly use the concepts of non-action and emptiness to generate life energy and improve the consciousness.

Huang Yuanji is also associated with the book "*Le Yu Tang*" which was written posthumously by his student. The special characteristic of Haung's Daoist meditation method is that it collects all previously existing Daoist theory and combines it into a cohesive and complete approach to using the ideas of Laozi to cultivate awareness and health. Previous Daoist writings tended to be much more arcane and dispersed, while Huang's method is clear and well planned out.

Huang emphasized quiet reflection, non-action, and being non-judgemental as the best way to attain the Dao and become enlightened.

Huang's school is often referred to as the Middle School and has a special emphasis on the use of meditation on the centre of the torso, rather than the lower *dantian* center in the abdomen.

Huang Yuanji's method represents the culmination of Daoist theory into a school that combines thoughts from every era of Daoist development and from other places such as Buddhism and Confucian ideals.

After the time of Huang Yuanji, Daoism again went into a lull, and by the end of the Qing dynasty in 1911, Daoism had descended into a confused amalgam of folk religions and superstition mostly popular among the Chinese peasant classes in rural areas such as Fujian, Shandong, Henan, and so on. Around this time, there were many invasions of China by foreign nations, and the country was also born into nationhood at the Republic of China, as lead by Sun Zhongshan and later by Jiang Jieshi (commonly known as Sun Yat Sen and Chiang Kaishek, in the western world).

With the birth of nationhood came the popularization of a "Chinese identity," and Jiang Jieshi was highly foundational in the documentation and popularization of martial arts as the Chinese national sport. Because of this backward looking attitude and the promotion of Chinese historical culture, there came to be a chance for the improvement of the situation of Daoism, which is the only Chinese indigenous religion to have ever achieved prominence in the minds of the Chinese people.

A man named Chen Yingning came forward as a scholar in Daoism who promoted the idea of "*Xian Xue*" or "The Study of God." His method of training used the fundamental ideas of Daoism, such as meditation on holism, in order to promote the idea that all religions share a common root in their search for immortality of the human spirit. Chen led a group of people in Shanghai who worked to create a secular and modern atmosphere in which they could gain benefit from Daoist practices. Although Chen died during the Cultural Revolution, his student Hu Haiya, a native of Zhejiang province, went on to establish himself as the president of the Beijing Daoist Research Association after it was reinstated after the Cultural Revolution.

Because of Hu Haiya's efforts, a great deal of academic research has been done on Daoism, and although the meditation tradition has not survived in many temples, it has been a staple of the Daoist tradition since the 1980s opening of China.

DAOISM TODAY

Daoism today exists both within the realm of religion and as something that normal people can study. The goals of people who practice religious Daoism are typically to gain favour with their gods and go to heaven after death, but the living tradition of Daoism is still contained within the early philosophical classics of Laozi and Zhuangzi, as well as the long and rich history of meditation documents left behind by past masters such as Lu Dongbin, Zhang Baoduan, Huang Yuanji, Chen Yingning, and so on.

Today in China, anyone who wishes to read Daoist classical documents may do so and most of the Daoist canon is available online. The amount of Daoist documents translated into English is still not complete, nor are all of the available translations truly representative of the genuine nature of Daoism, but it is still possible for non-Chinese speakers to study Daoism, and I hope that the ideas and practices presented in this book will assist you in your ongoing study.

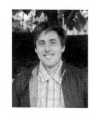

ABOUT THE AUTHOR

Growing up in a small Canada city, Robert Coons began his study of Daoism and Chinese culture at the age of eight. His father, long fascinated by Eastern spiritual traditions, gave Robert translations of Daoist books for children, and Robert Senior and Junior began studying Mandarin Chinese together at a local school.

Throughout Robert's childhood, he studied Asian martial arts and the leading ideas of other cultures and eras in world history. He later enrolled as a History major at the University of Guelph, where an influential professor helped guide his interest in Chinese culture and history. He also met Master Yang Hai, who is his current teacher in Daoism and the Chinese arts of Gongfu (kung fu) and Qi Gong (energy practice).

At the suggestion of his teacher, Robert went to China in search of a new perspective on martial arts. While living in Shanghai, he fell in love with Chinese traditional arts and culture. He has studied, among other things, Daoism, the internal martial arts, the study of tea culture, modern and ancient poetry and prose, calligraphy, brush painting, and pottery.

Robert currently resides both in Canada, where he runs a tea business and meditation club, and Henan, China, where he operates an English school and studies Chinese arts and culture. Robert also frequently gives classes on Daoism and martial arts in his home town of Guelph, Ontario, in Toronto, and elsewhere.

TAMBULI MEDIA

Excellence in Mind-Body Health & Martial Arts Publishing

Welcome to Tambuli Media, publisher of quality books on mind-body martial arts and wellness presented in their cultural context.

Our Vision is to see quality books once again playing an integral role in the lives of people who pursue a journey of personal development, through the documentation and transmission of traditional knowledge of mind-body cultures.

Our Mission is to partner with the highest caliber subject-matter experts to bring you the highest quality books on important topics of health and martial arts that are in-depth, well-written, clearly illustrated and comprehensive.

Tambuli is the name of a native instrument in the Philippines fashioned from the horn of a carabao. The tambuli was blown and its sound signaled to villagers that a meeting with village elders was to be in session, or to announce the news of the day. It is hoped that Tambuli Media publications will "bring people together and disseminate the knowledge" to many.

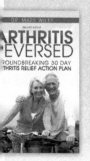
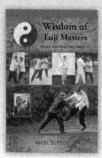
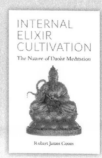
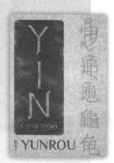

Spring House, PA
TambuliMedia.com

Made in the USA
Coppell, TX
31 December 2019

13937195R00088